The Hormone Connection

ENDING THE BATTLE BETWEEN THE SEXES

Dr. Patrick Flynn
"The Hormone Whisperer"

THE HORMONE CONNECTION: Ending the Battle Between the Sexes
Dr. Patrick Flynn, "*The Hormone Whisperer*"

For information, or to order additional copies, please contact:
TitleTown Publishing
P.O. Box 12093 | Green Bay, WI 54307-12093
920.737.8051 | www.titletownpublishing.com

Edited by *Erin Walton & Tracy C. Ertl*
Cover design by *The Wellness Way*
Prepared for publication by *Travis J. Vanden Heuvel*

PUBLISHER'S CATALOGING-IN-PUBLICATION DATA

Flynn, Patrick.
THE HORMONE CONNECTION: Ending the Battle Between the Sexes / Dr. Patrick Flynn. – 1st edition. Green Bay, WI : TitleTown Pub., c2017.

ISBN: 978-1-949042-00-9

Printed in the USA
10 9 8 7 6 5 4 3 2 1

ACKNOWLEDGMENTS:

A project like this doesn't just come together. Like everything else we do at The Wellness Way, "Team work makes the dream work!" I'd like to thank those who were a part of the team that brought this book in to reality.

Thank you to all who have helped make The Wellness Way a growing national brand; making a difference in the health of people around the world!

DEDICATION

To my beautiful bride, Christy:

I choose you.

INTRODUCTION

Allopathic, alternative, and every variation of each...there are many different approaches to healthcare. What is the Wellness Way Approach-how does it fit in?

We all know about the allopathic or mainstream approach to medicine. Go to the doctor, present symptoms, get a prescription or have surgery. Repeat. Alternative is similar, however, there are few in that world in agreement. In alternative or naturopathic medicine, you go to the doctor, present symptoms and treat with a natural remedy. Repeat.

And then there is The Wellness Way Approach. How do we fit into one of the boxes above? We don't. The Wellness Way Approach is a completely different way of looking at the body. When we have a patient come in with specific symptoms, we look deeper because we know that the body is sending messages. It is our job to put the puzzle pieces together to find the proper course of care for your unique and individual needs. We do this through specific tests, not standard procedures for the mass population. We have an approach, not a protocol. You are an individual and we treat you like one.

One thing that sets The Wellness Way Approach apart is

how we view the body as a collective whole. If you present one symptom, it may be reflective of a health challenge in a seemingly unrelated part of the body. However, we know that there are no unrelated organs or systems within the body. Everything is connected like an intricate Swiss watch.

The Swiss Watch Principle:

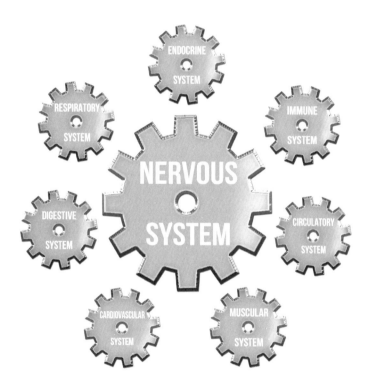

The human body is like a Swiss watch. It is very complex and composed of many, many parts. What would happen if the smallest gear stopped turning for just one moment?

Would you agree that it would affect the entire watch? Would it keep time properly? No, of course not.

Has anyone ever taken a medication for heart issues and later discovered the medication damaged their liver? The human body is like a Swiss watch with many gears all working together in harmony. You cannot treat one system (gear) without affecting them all.

For example, detoxification is a very important gear; but it is only one gear. There are others, the gear of proper nutrition, the gear of chiropractic care, the gear of proper mental health (such as the proper handling of stress), and the gear of proper hormone function and so on. If you have even one gear not working properly, you cannot be healthy.

If a person receives regular chiropractic care but eats fast food all the time and handles his/her stress poorly, this person will not be able to achieve true and complete health. Likewise, if a person takes care of proper nutrition and proper detoxification but neglects the gear of proper care of the nervous system, he or she will never achieve true health. We must have all the gears working together in harmony—this is true health.

To sum up, The Wellness Way looks at each individual patient as unique. We look at the whole "watch" not just a part of it. We address the cause (or causes) of ill health, not just the symptoms.

In this same way, a person's male or female hormones can affect all parts of their lives and marriage. With that in mind, let's dive in to *End The Battle Between The Sexes!*

CHAPTER 1

Eighteen years ago, I fell in love with a beautiful woman. I mean, I fell, and I fell hard. On the second date, she told me "I'm going to marry you someday" and I told her "You're right!" Christy and I spent the first two weeks of our relationship sharing our hearts and what we each wanted for our lives. She shared her dreams; I shared my vision and direction. We discussed the family we wanted to have, where we wanted to live, our passions and goals. We also shared how we would raise our children and the ways we wanted to make a difference in the world. Remember, we were young. I was just finishing up chiropractic school. During the second week of our relationship, I went to her house and found her on the floor in fetal position, crying. She was sobbing. My first thought – – c'mon guys, you know this feeling--"Oh no! What did I do?!"

I hadn't done anything. She was sobbing because she had gotten her cycle that day. She was actually crying because she was in so much pain. Christy started telling me the story of her health history. This was a history I didn't know about with female hormone problems she had been dealing with for years. To go along with the physical challenges, she shared

11

with me that she had been told she may not be able have kids; she may be infertile. If Christy were ever to conceive a child, she most likely would not be able to carry a pregnancy to term. She even went as far as to say maybe we shouldn't be together. Now, I had a decision to make. While we had been sharing our hearts in that fantastic first two weeks of our relationship, I had shared with her I wanted a big family. So, I had a choice to make right there. Do I stay with her or do I leave her? I'm not kidding when I told you I had completely fallen head over heels for that beautiful woman. Do I chalk this up as a set back? Or, do I choose to use it as a set up for one of the greatest gifts God has ever given me?

Because I loved Christy and we had a future in front of us we both clearly wanted, the choice was obvious. The choice was her; it was us. I engulfed myself into the study of female hormones. I devoured everything I could find, every research article, every study, everything. I spoke with other doctors I respected, people who had been my instructors while I was in school and others who had a mindset to look at things differently. I wanted to see multiple perspectives and put the pieces together. I studied female hormones like a fanatic. The best answers I found were crap. All I could think was: *"Man, they have it all wrong!"* I knew this didn't line up with what I had been taught in school. I couldn't settle for crap. I knew there was more to it. I had to keep digging and look at it from a different approach.

We had obstacles. Every decision you make will have obstacles. The question is, will you overcome the obstacles to get to the end you want? First of all, Christy felt discouraged by the medical method of handling her condition. She was not getting any better and wasn't getting any answers that would actually help her to get better and healthy. You see, she had been to some of the best specialists she could go to. She was definitely ready and willing to try something different. Of course, Christy had fears and doubts and would have to trust *me* – a guy she just met – on this journey! I may have been a new doctor, but I was convinced a woman's body was meant to have babies. All bodies are created for homeostasis, health and function. That was more than any other doctor had offered her. I chose to look at things differently and not settle for the answers she had been given. This unfamiliar approach was foreign to both of our families and as a result caused stress and struggles within our relationships. We chose to stay with it no matter what, including all the criticisms when living under a microscope.

Do you want to see the result and impact our decision to pursue Christy's health made? We have four amazing daughters. Yes, I have *FOUR* daughters. You can all pray for me now.

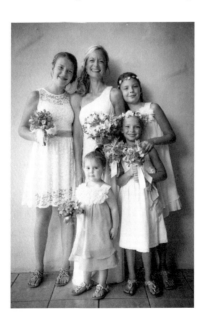

There's another huge impact from that original choice to pursue health. One I hadn't known at the time when Christy and I chose to build a future together, but a result that has impacted men, women, and children all over the world. It was a change of thought process. I had to look at things from a different approach and not just settle for the "one size fits all" method the medical world uses. The Wellness Way wouldn't be where it is today if I hadn't chosen Christy and her unique health. Actually, a huge national company impacting thousands of people a year around the world would not exist if I hadn't chosen my wife. This pivotal change of thought process impacted my wife and created the opportunity for us to have a family with those four amazing daughters. Now I'm using our experience to help families all over the world. Do you see what I mean when I say your choices will have an impact? It all started with a change in thought process.

In my research, I found the first contribution to the study of hormones ever recorded happened in 1050 B.C. by a Chinese emperor. He had two wooden troughs made. He had young men urinate in one, then let the urine dehydrate. He took the other trough and had ladies urinate into it and let that one dehydrate as well. He found that there was a film left at the bottom of the troughs. They took a spicy, gummy substance and rubbed it into the bottom of the troughs. The emperor ate the one that had come from the trough of the young men. The one from the trough of the young women, he fed to his wives. What they found was that they were happier, had less infections, lived longer, and the women were less moody. I can see it now, some of your faces are like, "that's disgusting!" 3,000 years later, guess what the number one form of hormone treatment is for women? Horse urine. *Preg*nant *Mar*e Ur*ine*. Now, ladies, think for just a moment. Do the ladies you know resemble a horse at all? I'm not joking!

I have some simple multiple-choice questions for you. Don't worry, I'll help you along with the answers. Would you agree in the past 2,000 years we have more hospitals? Yes or yes? More doctors? Yes or yes? Spend more money on health care? And today, that is still the best thing to offer women, especially if they are over the age of 40. Horse urine.

I had to keep studying, so I kept reading and researching. The stuff I found was mind blowing. Let me ask you a question. If you have a daughter, when she gets to her teenage years, she's going to go through a change in life, correct? It's called puberty and it's natural. It happens to every young woman. Yet, there are times when the medical approach looks for "solutions" to these natural phases of life.

Here was an interesting article I found. Horse hormone given to young women to stop them from having a menstrual cycle. I found this article in a very popular "health" magazine. The article starts: "Sick of your period? Get rid of it!" I read the article and thought, *maybe this is the thing, maybe they have it right. Perhaps women don't need a cycle.* At the University of Florida Health Sciences Medical School, with the assistance of medication, doctors have now agreed that cycles are optional. But only with the help of a medication. I started to research this idea further and I found that doctors believe there is no medical reason to menstruate. Ever. I had to read what the medication does to make this possible, because this obviously wasn't a natural process. The prescribed medication causes the uterine lining to harden so you won't have a period anymore. However, underneath everything still works. What do you think this causes the uterus to do? Like a balloon, it gets bigger and bigger until it actually explodes. The doctors agreed this is not dangerous, however, it may be inconvenient. Ladies, if your uterus explodes, is that a little bit more than inconvenient?

I spent time reading thousands of articles by the "best doctors in their field" and this was the best I could find. This was the only thing they had for my wife. After all my reading and research, after seeing hundreds of women a year for 18 years, I can speak with great confidence on one thing. You want to know what it is? I thank God, every day, I don't have a vagina. Every day. Guys, we are pretty lucky and have it pretty easy. We really do. I also started to realize women didn't understand their own bodies. My wife at that time was 23 years old and had no clue. Many women today have no clue what is going on with their bodies. They don't understand men and their hormones, but neither do men understand their own hormones nor those of their partners. I'm going to take you on a path, so you can understand how I began to understand these hormones and functions and how we are able to convey this approach in offices all over the country. To take you on this journey and bring understanding, I need to get you to do what I did and learn to think differently. I will set the stage for the rest of the book. I'm also certain I'll offend most of you through this process and step on some toes. That's okay. I'm more concerned with speaking truth and reality than making friends.

Think about some of the statistics we see daily. Now versus any time in history, do we have more or less heart disease? More or less cancer? More or less fertility problems? If we keep on that same thinking, most of you will have the same situations as everybody else. Just because something is common does not mean it's normal. I want to offend you so that you will start thinking differently. To get you to think differently, I have to come up with an altered approach. That is The Wellness Way Approach.

When I have someone come into my office, I prefer to meet with couples. It makes the most sense. When both partners hear the message from the same source, there will be less confusion and we will be able to communicate more clearly. Also, it will help the person we are most focusing on to have a support person. Often there are real and practical steps the support person can do to help our patient. I'm aware that most of the healthcare decisions (approximately 95%) are made by wives and most of the people who pick up this book first will be women. However, I'm going to take the approach through this book as if I were speaking to both of you, a husband and a wife, in my office. If the wife gets this approach and she shares it with her husband, they will start an amazing process of getting healthy and having a happier marriage together. If you are single, you only have to read half the book to understand yourself, but I would recommend reading the whole thing if you ever plan to be married, or care to understand the opposite sex!

CHAPTER 2

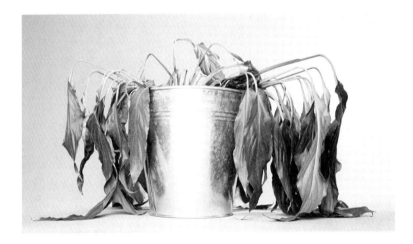

W hat do you think this plant needs? Water. Why didn't you say drugs or surgery? Why didn't you say horse hormones? You've been taught better to take care of a rotten plant than your own body. That's how troubling medicine is. We're taught to listen to the doctor. However, most of those doctors are clueless when it comes to hormones. They don't know how to measure them, they don't know how to take care of them, and they don't know how to get them back to normal. There's one set of clinics that does know how-The Wellness Way.

Anyone who knows me, knows that I love to create analogies and use them frequently. Why? We've all sat with doctors, looked at them, they've looked at us, and we made sure that we were listening. Then when we left the appointment and thought, *"what in the world did they just say?"*

The doctor sounded very smart but didn't connect with you. You had no clue what you were doing, and you were taking him or her on blind faith. Let me give you an example. Before I sit down with a woman, I go through the list of medications she is taking. If a woman is taking something like Premarin, I ask her if she has an affinity for carrots. I'm trying to get her to think differently. When they look at me like I'm crazy, I say "Well, you are putting horse urine into your body and they like carrots and sugar cane, so I was just wondering." Women get downright mad when they learn what their doctor has really prescribed to them! And they should get mad. Would you agree that if a woman has been given a horse hormone and doesn't know it, she should be mad? Absolutely. I don't have a problem with someone taking something as long as they know what they are taking, what it is doing, why they are taking it, for how long they will be taking it, and all the effects that go along with that plan.

This is the analogy that has set the foundation for everything since I started. It sets the basis for every patient we see at The Wellness Way. I believe if you understand this simple analogy, you will understand which doctor to use. Some of you are reading this book because you are frustrated with your doctor. You are downright mad and won't go back. I'm not saying you shouldn't go back, I'm saying you should know *why* and *when* to go back. By the time we are done here, I want you to be able to have a clearer understanding, know what you know, and believe what you believe. No fence sitting allowed.

Firemen and Carpenters

Let's say you've been out for a nice dinner with your family and you get home to find your house on fire. Who is the best professional to handle this situation? A fireman. Why wouldn't you call your dentist? Doesn't he have a hose? You're thinking, *"Doc, that's a stupid question!"* Well, it's a stupid question because you know that if he showed up with his tools and his hose he could get himself killed. The fireman is the best trained professional to handle the situation.

So, let's walk through the scenario. The firetruck pulls up and the firemen basically have two tools to work with; hoses and axes. With the ax, the firefighter runs up to your house where he crashes your door in and then smashes the windows. The guy with the hose then runs in and starts spraying the inside of your house. Simple question, when the water he sprays hits the pictures of your kids, what does it do to them? The wall? What does it do to the carpet? The fire department has been there about 15 minutes and what have they done to your house so far? You are standing there, and you are grateful for all the different ways they have *destroyed* your home. You are grateful because you've been trained to be! All you'll have left is a burned-out shell of your home, and you are grateful. Even though they caused massive destruction you are not mad. Why? This is their job. But, can you live in that house? Is it toxic? Could it kill you? Let's remember, the fire department has done a good job and has done everything they were supposed to do with the knowledge and tools they have to work with.

A time will come when you've got to get back into your house. Who is the best professional to call now? The carpenter. Imagine the carpenter shows up while the fire department is still there. The carpenter sees a mess! He has to rip out walls and carpet and bring in the materials he needs to rebuild the house. Which person is right? Both, based on the specific need of the house at the specific time. If the carpenter shows up to the house while it's on fire, he looks like what? He looks like an idiot! If he shows up with his tools of a hammer, nails, and lumber he looks like an idiot. Vice versa, if the fire department shows up and tries to rebuild the house with an ax and a hose, they look like idiots. Would you agree? I'm not being mean, but based on the need, you have to know which professional to call.

If you understand that example, you understand how healthcare should be run today. If you are having a stroke or heart attack, with the education you know that I have, should I run into your kitchen and grab a knife and see if I can help you? No, because I'd look like what? I'd look like an idiot! We need to call someone who is the best professional to save your life. Who are we going to call? We're going to call 911. For the purposes of the analogy, let's call medicine the fire department. They're going to take you to the hospital and use their axes and hoses on you. Here's where some confusion comes in. When they put the hose into your arm and start pumping the medicine into your body, is it good for your body? Some say yes, and some say no. Let's go back to the example. When the fire department sprays water on the walls, is it good for the walls? You have to answer the question that was asked. I didn't ask if it saved your life. I didn't ask if it put out the fire. I asked if it was good for your body. If you look at the back of the medication bottle and the inserts, there are numerous warnings and negative side effects, and they are definitely *not* good for your body. The manufacturer presents this information. I'm not saying it's not needed, I'm just asking if it's good for you.

Now, let's say the medication didn't work. They only have one other tool; the ax. Could you possibly die from that surgery? Ok, can we come to an agreement? Could we agree that if you are having a heart attack, you may need drugs or surgery to stay alive? Even if they aren't necessarily good for your body, they are what is needed at the time to save the body from dying.

Let's go back to my wife. Did they give her medications when she presented her symptoms? If they are the fire department, they start with medication. The challenges my wife was dealing with would eventually develop into cancer. Then it would be time for the ax. They would tell her to have her uterus removed via hysterectomy. She went to some top specialists; but their way of thinking was the fire department. Do you follow me?

Let's look at the difference. Can you guess the number one reason why people have gone to the doctors in recent years? High blood pressure. Everybody knows someone with high blood pressure. Can someone die from high blood pressure? Yes or yes? Do I have any problem with the fire department's approach using ACE inhibitors, channel blockers or Lasix? No, they save people's lives. But after the life has been saved, after all the warm thank yous to the doctors and nurses, do they ever sit down with you and discuss why you've had the heart attack or stroke? Do they help you get your body back to healthy? Really, do you think they *really* work to get you back to healthy? They may suggest a bland diet that feels like a death sentence and an occasional walk, but are they helping you to rebuild for a long and vibrant life? Can you rebuild a house with an ax and a hose? No, you can only put out a fire. Can you get your body back to normal with drugs or surgery? No, you can't. Today, we have fire department doctors. The Wellness Way Approach is the carpenter approach. I want to know what triggered your fire. The Wellness Way helps our patients to repair the weak spots where fires can start, rebuild where fires have been, and best of all prevent any possible fires so that you can live that long and vibrant life!

When Christy presented me with these problems, I figured out what triggered *her* fires and how to rebuild *her* house. That's how we have four daughters today.

Let's take a look from another example in my office. What's the number one medication given for high blood pressure today? Many people take the medication Atenolol. Atenolol can save a life. I'm not saying it can't. But let's not forget a negative side effect is extreme fatigue. I had a woman come in with female hormone problems as well as extreme fatigue and thought I could help her. I looked at her medication list and told her I couldn't help her unless I found what was causing her to have high blood pressure. If I didn't find the cause, she could never remove this medication-which was causing the fatigue! Do you see the difference in thought process? The firefighter approach would have put her on something to change her energy level, correct? Could that have worked? Yes, but now you've added another medication. The average person today is taking 4-7 prescribed medications. If you watch TV or read ads in magazines, you will see medications competing over who can put out the fire faster. But they missed the point. I just ask a different question which is what caused the fire in the first place? The key comes back to finding the trigger.

People often say "Doc, I get it! I know what you do now! Instead of taking the medical fire department approach, you are the alternative approach."

Now, let me tell you something. That thinking is just as wrong as the first approach. Can a person take magnesium and vitamin B shots and other natural things to lower their blood pressure? Yes, they can, but it's still the wrong way to think about the situation. All they are doing is using natural things to put out the fire instead of the medical things. People often say these things have no negative side effects. After 18 years I found the number one side effect associated with this kind of therapy. It's called a thinner pocketbook. Let me show you why. Between the alternative and the medical, which one will fail first?

Imagine at one of my seminars I brought in a whole bag of Viagra and gave each one of the guys a dose. What's going to happen over the next four hours even if they didn't need it? None of those guys would stand up. Do you want to know why? That medication is going to work. It can force your body to work even if you don't need or want it to. The natural thing will always fail first because it can't force the body to do something. The good news is that's why there are no negative side effects, but at one point it will stop working.

You've seen this situation a million times. The latest and greatest "miracle" fad hits the newsstands and TV talk shows. Everyone needs to jump on the bandwagon, self-diagnose and self-treat with these natural "remedies." It doesn't work for everybody and all of a sudden, this herb, mineral or vitamin that is so vital, powerful and beneficial gets a bad rap because people don't know what their specific health challenge is nor how to really take care of themselves. There's no guidance.

Not everything will work for everybody. Is your body the same as another person's, even if you are related? No, it's very different. That's why The Wellness Way Approach is unique to each individual. The Wellness Way Approach knows that while two people may be related and while their houses may have some similarities, they are different and daily living in each house is different. Our approach is quite simple. I tested my wife from a different mindset. What triggered *her* fire and how do I rebuild *her* body? I didn't just balance my wife's hormones to get her pregnant four times, I got her body healthy. It's perfectly normal for a healthy woman to have a baby. That's a positive side effect!

Our motto at the Wellness Way is *"We don't guess… we test!"* We don't test for fires, we test for what could trigger a fire and how to rebuild the house in such a way as to prevent that fire from ever occurring again. I know you didn't pick up this book to read about hormone issues. You really didn't. You were looking for something else, something that seems elusive.

What is health, anyway?

At my seminars, I ask people to raise their hand if they want to be healthy, if they want healthy kids, healthy parents and healthy in-laws. The funny thing is very few people can tell me what "healthy" is. I hear a variety of answers and even a few responses of "I don't know." It makes sense. We've been taught about fires our whole lives such as cancer, diabetes, heart disease and all the others you see in drug commercials. Everybody wants to be healthy, but we know very little about it. That's why so many people are sick today.

Here's another question I ask people about health. What are three things that make you healthy? I already know what they will say. We've been conditioned in so many ways to do what we've been told to do. Food, exercise and sleep. Just about everyone agrees these three things make you healthy. It's yet another reason why people are so sick. These three things have very little to do with *making* you healthy.

You know people who never eat well, never exercise, smoke every day and live to be 100 years old. George Burns lived to be 100 and we all know that he was very open with his cigars and martinis. Then you have people who simply come in contact with second-hand smoke and get cancer. Ladies, you know you hate those women who eat four donuts in the morning, never exercise and are thin.

You may be confused and thinking food, exercise and sleep aren't important for you. I didn't say that. I asked you if that is where health *comes f*rom. They are very important to your health, but they aren't where health comes from. Just like when we talked about the house on fire, is putting the water on the walls good for the walls? We need to start thinking differently. If I hadn't learned to think differently, my beautiful bride would never have had those four beautiful babies.

What's my story? How did all this start? I grew up in a small town called Twin Bridge near Crivitz, in northern Wisconsin. We were a very poor family and I was a very sick child. I was labeled in third grade as a troubled child after I got so irritated I beat up a kid. The counselor told my mom I was a bad kid and I would probably end up in jail. I didn't realize my health conditions were causing my brain to go 100 miles per hour and my skin to feel like it was crawling. At one point, I had a bad allergic reaction and was put on a medication.

My brain started to calm down-even though the reason the medication was prescribed had nothing to do with my brain. The purpose of the medication was to calm my immune system. In the process of calming my immune system, my brain calmed down. Today, we know why this happened. Most of our immune system is in our gut and half of the neurotransmitters for our brain are made there as well. Think about that. 90% of our serotonin is made in our gut. That's why food brings us so much emotion.

I went to the Crivitz library and started my research. I found a book that explained how the immune system works. I still have that book today. I started to read and research that book and learn what health is. There I was, 13 years old and asking what health is 29 years ago and they were clueless; they are even more clueless today.

We still use the definition of "health" today as it was defined in the 1950's:

A state of optimal physical and social wellbeing and not merely the absence of diseases (or what we call fires).

Let me give you an example from my office. I had a nurse practitioner from a local hospital visit me. She thought she had some hormone problems. We went through our normal exam. I took some x-rays and I saw a tumor. You know what I told her to do? I told her to go back to the hospital and check to make sure she wasn't going to die. Why? Can I rebuild the house if you are dead? No. They took a biopsy and decided since it wasn't going to grow they'd just monitor it each year. That was the decision between her and her fire department type doctor. Let's say it was cancer and could have killed her. If they pulled it out, did they extend her life? Possibly. Did they make her healthy? No. Within 2-5 years we all know what happens in this story. When you tell people from the "natural" side of healthcare, the reason we live so long today is medicine, they tend to freak out. Drugs and surgery have done a good job of keeping us alive. They are doing their job. But we are still sick as dogs because they don't make us healthy.

I don't like that definition of health, so I created one that I think is more accurate. Here's the definition of health we use at The Wellness Way:

A condition of wholeness in which all the organs are functioning 100% of the time.

Let's go back to the three healthy choices of food, exercise and sleep. If I cut my finger and my body is functioning well, it will heal. If my body is not functioning well, there are conditions where I could bleed to death. If I cut my finger, do I have to eat a healthy sandwich for it to heal? Do I have to take a nap? Jump on a treadmill? Do you see the difference? Those choices are good to help rebuild your house, but that is not where health comes from. All health is about function. For the rest of the book we'll take the carpenter perspective and apply it to how hormones are supposed to function properly.

Dr. Patrick Flynn

Intro to hormones, moderation and stress.

The number one cause of hormone problems, especially in women, is stress. I'm going to define it for you, so we are all clear what exactly stress is. First let's start with who stresses out more, men or women? Women. Who causes women the most stress? I'll prove it to you that *men* are one of the biggest contributors to illness on the planet today. I'm not joking! Hang with me guys, it gets better. I really want you to understand this; let's define what stress is.

Stress: a physical...

What does a chiropractor really do? Remove physical stress. You may be thinking, *"No Doc, my chiropractor makes my pain go away."* Have you ever gotten adjusted and the pain did not go away? Let me raise my hand first. Have you ever gotten adjusted and your headache did not go away? Let me raise my hand first. The point is, because today we are so dominant in the fire department medical system, we define all professionals within that perspective. That's not true. Chiropractors just do one thing. They are the carpenter doctor that removes that physical stress. But usually that's not the only stress. Let's go on.

...or psychological stimulus that can lead to and produce mental or physiological reactions that may lead to illness.

Technically speaking, stress is a disruption to homeostasis which may be triggered by alarming experiences either real or perceived. 80% of the stuff you worry about never happens. Statistically men are less sick than women. Do you know why? Because most of the time we just don't care. All the ladies are laughing because you know it's true. The guys are not laughing because they know they're in trouble now.

Stress is a physical, chemical or emotional *thing*. Yes, you can get adjusted if you want to remove the physical stresses. I had to do that for my wife to help her remove some of those stressors. Chemicals. Can you eat chemicals? Yes, you can. Most people eat a lot of them, not at my house, but a lot of people do. That's why The Wellness Way doctors are so focused on what you eat. Let me illustrate in a way that will most likely offend a few folks.

Grandma has told you some very idiotic things. Now, you're thinking, *"Doc, are you calling my grandma an idiot?"* Well, grandma may not be an idiot. But, she has most likely told you some idiotic things based on her perspective of "healthy," the emotional influences of food, and how she shows her love for you. Let me explain. Grandma comes to you after you've started to eat healthy. She brings a plate of chocolate chip cookies with all the junk ingredients and she sweetly says, "Here honey, I have some cookies for you" and you say, "No thank you, Grandma, I'm not going to eat those." And Grandma says, "Everything is good in moderation!" Grandma's perspective is idiotic. Your body doesn't know if something is good or not. It knows if something is inflammatory and creates stress or if it is not inflammatory. It doesn't know moderation. Remember, food and eating is one of the most emotional things we do.

Let me give you an example. Here's some good health advice for married couples; don't have sex for a week. Now the guy will be kinda mad, the gal will be just fine. Right? But here's another angle. If I tell that same couple to fast for three days, they'll both hate me. Food carries a lot of emotional influence.

Just to help understand this point, I've defined moderation for us:

"Moderation is your emotional justification to eat something bad for you."

It's just emotional, that's all it is.

I want you to think about this. You can get adjusted and pull all the chemicals out of your body and eat organic but guess what is 10x more disruptive to health than anything else. Mental stress. It will kill you. All doctors are taught this.

So, back to my study. I started to study women. I studied why they stressed out so much. I polled women 18 years ago and I still ask them today. What do women care about? Everything. But what are the top three things that cause the most stress?

WOMEN	MEN
1. **Men**	1. **Work**
2. **Children**	2. **Sex**
3. **Weight**	3. **Kids**

Top Stressors by Gender

Here's where I'm going to offend a bunch of women. Women, it's very clear where we are on your stress list. Ladies, where are you on our stress list? You're not. There's only one way you can stress out a guy, ladies. I'm going to show you there's a biological reason why. Ladies, if you understand this, you can make this man chase you and love you for the rest of your life. But because you don't understand this one little thing, you think he's a pig. He's perverted and disgusting. No. You just don't understand the man, and our society has been trying to tell men they need to be more "nice" and "sensitive". Let's take a good look at that man, what makes him a real, healthy man and how to keep him that way.

Some Things to Think About in a New Way

CHAPTER 3

Before we start this chapter, I know I need to add some flowers here for the ladies, so you don't assume I'm a jerk. Who am I kidding, I'm a guy. I think like a guy. I have learned to understand the differences between a man and a woman. I'm not coming down on women, *but*, I am going to call things as I have seen them for years in my office. Remember, we are going to think differently here, and you chose to marry a man, or at the very least you live in a society where men exist. You have to accept him as he was created to be. I'm not going to contribute to the current political and social perception that men need to become sissies so as not to be jerks. Men have been created as they are for very real and good purposes. Just like everything else on the planet, things meant for good can be twisted, disrupted and misunderstood with a little help from humans. Welcome to life on planet Earth. Just understand, I have learned the best way to teach something is to speak it like it is. I'm not a jerk, ladies, but I am also not a sissy. I'm a man who cares more about speaking truth than keeping the peace and making friends.

I'm a man who happens to understand a lot about hormones, both male and female. Stick with me.

Let's start with the guys' cycle. It's quite simple, but I'm going to reveal something that has eluded men and women for generations. Ladies, you don't understand your guy's cycle and the hormones involved so you don't understand your man. We're actually pretty simple to understand once you see it. Don't worry, men are completely oblivious to the fact that there is a cycle and the hormones involved, and it's his. Actually, he just doesn't much care, and soon, we'll all understand why. I know how he feels. I operate just like all the other guys.

In my seminars, I often ask women what they want in a man. I hear things like:

compassionate
kind
a good listener
thoughtful
gentle

Ladies, I think I may have found the problem. You aren't looking for a man, you are looking for a woman. When you understand the basic biological differences in our hormones, you understand the simple fact remains that men and women are very different to their core. No matter what the politically correct media and Hollywood would have us think today, we aren't the same and it has little to do with the clothes we prefer to wear. A man can't be a woman and a woman can't be a man. There will be so much less confusion in this world once we get over the notion of "gender confusion."

Have you ever seen little boys and girls play together? They get along just fine. Their hormones are quite similar and consistent. Then, that magical time called puberty comes about and turns the whole relationship upside down. They don't know if they love each other or hate each other. Throwing two cats in a burlap sack would be more peaceful than watching the interaction between two pubescent adolescents of the opposite sex try to interact. What happened? They still have the same genes and phenotypes, but something has changed, and it's changed dramatically. Their hormones have started to change their childhood bodies into bodies of a man and a woman. They may not be able to describe or explain it, but they can sure feel it—and so can everyone else around them.

What's the one hormone that really makes us guys who we are? The one we always want to say with a little bit of "GRRRR". Testosterone. It makes us men. Testosterone at a young age is pretty low, it's supposed to be. When that young man hits puberty, it rises significantly. Here's the cool thing. How long does testosterone stay high in a man? Forever. This is the biggest mistake and number one lie about men's health you've learned from the fire department medical system. People believe that as a man ages and gets older, his testosterone will decrease. No, it does not, that's a lie. Any doctor that tells you that is an idiot and doesn't know what they are talking about. Guys, and their ladies, don't know how to take care of themselves so their house continues to rot, and their testosterone levels drop. Testosterone doesn't naturally fall; it falls because of another fire in the house. It is possible to keep a guy's testosterone normal his whole life, and it's simple. That's the whole cycle. Testosterone low, puberty, testosterone high for the rest of his life. Ladies, pay attention, I'm going to teach you how to keep your man's hormones normal in a way that will cost you virtually nothing.

What does testosterone do?

One of the obvious things testosterone does is cause physical changes. It gives us energy, it gives us muscle development, and it gives us our sexual drive. A man's testosterone cycle is highest in the morning. Ladies, you know how you can tell. If you don't believe me, tomorrow morning before he wakes up lift the covers and if he's a healthy boy, something's going to be awake before he is…and he has no control over it. There's nothing wrong with him. His testosterone is normal, so his body responds. He has no physical control over that morning erection. Remember that bit of info and don't shame him for it. Thank God you have a healthy man.

Hormones also change us mentally. Testosterone gives a man great confidence. Every healthy man, regardless of his age, thinks he's amazing. Right, ladies? Do you ever see your husband in front of a mirror? He's flexing and checkin' himself out. It doesn't matter how old he is. Testosterone gives us this great confidence. Ladies, you don't have the amount of testosterone we do so you tend to down play it. When a man can be confident and unashamed, that's healthy. Let him be a man. You need to stop putting him down for his confidence. Encourage that boy! That's normal and healthy.

The second function of testosterone is to keep him motivated and driven. Testosterone is *why* he does what he does; it is a very driving hormone. If somebody were to break into your house tonight, which of you will get up to chase the criminal? Your man will, why? Because when testosterone rises, it makes him aggressive. Ladies, you like that; until you create the same reaction in him as if a criminal who broke into your house. Remember the big steroid hormone craze of the 80's? It was a craze alright. What happens when you give a man a synthetic testosterone to supplement his natural testosterone? He will go crazy with aggression.

Here's one piece of relationship advice you can both thank me for. Imagine you've just had what I like to call "an intense moment of fellowship," some may call it a fight. Ladies, your hormones make you want to talk. Don't talk to him. He's not going to die; leave him alone. He'll cool off and come back with a much more level head and be able to have the conversation you want to have. Many devastating and mean things are said by husbands when they are mad. When he relaxes, that testosterone returns to normal. When you are both able to speak calmly, he always says "honey, I didn't mean it that way." And he didn't. He was responding to the rise in testosterone due to the rise in tensions in the situation. He can't control the rise in testosterone. I'm not saying he shouldn't control his response. When his testosterone rises, it tells him to kill whatever is sitting in front of him. If that's you, it's a bad day. In no way am I justifying the horrific domestic abuse caused by disgusting men who are out of control. I'm explaining what a rapid rise of testosterone causes in the brain.

Testosterone also makes him very single task focused. Once you realize where it comes from, it's very obvious to see in various ways throughout his life. Ladies, your guy can only think about one thing at a time. Consider them professionally-guys tend to climb the ladder of success quickly. Men are driven because they can focus on just one thing at a time. Testosterone tells the guy's brain to go after whatever he sees.

Think about that fact in terms of relationships. Ladies, do you think testosterone tells a guy:

"be nice to the girl"

"romance the girl"

"get her flowers"

NO! It tells him to "chase the girl!" See, you want us to be like you. But we don't have the same hormones you do, so we can't be like you. It doesn't make us bad or perverted, it makes us men. What most likely attracted you to that guy was the opposite of your hormones. He pursued you with a clear purpose and was relentless in that pursuit. Today, politically, we think men and women are capable of being the same. They are not. They never *could* be; their biology would never allow it to happen.

In the evening, a man's testosterone starts to decrease a little bit. His ability to listen and focus on his lady increases. He's also more agreeable, passive and low key. Ladies, let me tell you step one in how to win with your man. If you try to tell your husband to do something in the morning—you might as well have not told him at all. Let me give you an example.

You ask him to take out the garbage. He's laser focused on the day ahead of him. He's not really listening to you and he leaves. When he closes the door and walks out, the garbage is still left there. The lady in this situation creates perceived stress, and let's be honest, some insane reasons for eight hours about why he didn't take out the garbage. We've all been there. He's forgotten about it the minute he left the door, he didn't hear you and you stew all day, either mad or with hurt feelings. You end up creating a lot of stress and actually make yourself sick with this anger due to the imaginary reasons you've created in your mind. When he comes home, he has been laser focused, energetic and aggressive all day and you've been angry and frustrated all day. Your first response is to argue about why he didn't take out the garbage like you so sweetly asked him. His response, "No you didn't!" and off to the races with another fight. Ladies, understand, if you want to talk to your man and have his focused attention, don't do it in the morning. This will save so many fights. If his testosterone is normal, he's already in high gear and not hearing you. I know some call this selective hearing. He's really not trying to ignore you; his brain is just focused with the morning dose of testosterone he naturally needs to make it through the day.

The Man Zone

We've discussed the fact testosterone rises drastically during puberty and remains high his whole life. I want your man in the Man Zone all the time, that's normal.

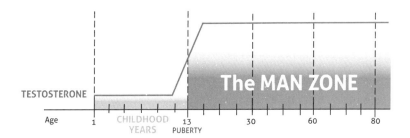

What do you think is the most common challenge with men in the Man Zone? I hear ladies whine, "But Doc, you

41

don't understand, my husband wants sex every day!" My response is simple "that's a good healthy boy!" Are guys perverted? Are they disgusting? Nope, sexually driven? Yes. And guess what. Men, you're a real man. Be proud of it! Women, you married him because you wanted a man. That's part of the package.

We want those guys to stay in the Man Zone. If they don't, they'll get very sick. I'm going to teach you ladies how to build his testosterone and keep your man healthy. You can help him increase his testosterone, so you can get him to do virtually anything you want. I'm going to give you a *To Do List*. Don't worry, I'm not putting all the work on you. You get off easy. The men will have two *To Do Lists*. Don't worry, they can handle it. They have testosterone to motivate them.

#1 Show the Boy

Let me explain this a bit. Ladies you have to stop dressing like a woman devoted to celibacy before you go to bed at night. I'll let that sink in for a minute. Your Snuggie is not sexy. Flannel is for children and grandma. We can only go after what we can see.

I can already hear the arguments, "Doc, when we were first married, my boobs were way up here, and now they're way down here."

Ladies, let me tell you something; we will hold them right where they belong. We will, we're nice like that. We don't care. The only person who cares is you. We're big picture thinkers. Most of the time we are completely unaware of the details. You know that. It works here too. Let me share a story to illustrate this point.

When I turned 16 I bought my first car for $150. It was a royal blue 1978 Pinto station wagon with no muffler. It was a chick magnet. I used to pull up to Crivitz High School and lean up next to my car like James Dean without the cigarette. I was so proud. You know why? Because it was mine. Ladies, that's the way a healthy man thinks about you. Just ask any man if he wants to see his wife naked tonight. If he's a healthy boy and a real man, you know he will. He doesn't see the stretch marks, the extra few pounds and the sag you do. He sees his wife, and he's dang proud of her. That should reduce a lot of emotional stress for you ladies. If you know how this works, you can get him to do whatever you want—and you'll both be happier!

#2 Talk to the Boy

You may think you talk to him all the time. But you talk to him in a way that feeds *your* hormones. Right now, we are talking about *his* hormones. There is a way you can talk to your man to get him to do what you want him to do all day. All you have to do tomorrow morning is grab that aggressive boy before he leaves for work and whisper into his ear, "Honey, tonight is going to be a good night!" What do you think your husband will be thinking about all day long?

When he gets home, he's going to get the kids ready for bed, and do the dishes. He's going to do everything he needs to do because his testosterone has been stimulated to. You have a motivated man. That's how a man works.

If you don't want to do that, some other woman will. If you don't talk to him the way he needs to be talked to and you don't show him what he needs to see, some other girl will. It won't be intentional on his part. He'll be at work someday and when that pretty girl walks by and says something to him or dresses in a way that shows him a little more than you have been, he can't help but be stimulated. Either you accept how this works, or you can be just as unhappy as the majority of marriages are today. We get wrapped up in the thought that men and women are created the same. They are not. Has the divorce rate in the last 20 years increased or decreased? That seems to be about the timing as to when we started trying to force men to be more like women. They are what they are. When we accept that men and women were created a specific and different way we'll all be able to get along much better. I know I keep hammering this point, but so does the media and our culture. Once we accept reality we'll be able to move on from this. Until then, we'll have to continue to hammer this point over and over.

#3 Don't Feed the Boy

I know men like #1 and #2 but they're not going to like #3.

As your husband gains too much weight, his testosterone will convert to another type of hormone, estrogens. That's why breast cancer is second to prostate cancer in men today. As their breasts, and the rest of them, get larger, their hormones convert to estrogens. Fat does a very good job of producing and storing estrogens making those men become more female like in hormones. Estrogens rising too high are currently the only known cause of breast cancer. A few times after taking a man's blood work, I have had him fast for 72 hours and his testosterone would rise anywhere from 25-40%. Men need to fast. I like to recommend a 72-hour fast every three months to help with testosterone levels. Ladies, sometimes you may have to put the kibosh on him and tell him he needs to take a break for a couple of days. Remember how I told you about foods and emotions? It's just as true for guys as it is for women.

#4 Capture the Boy's Mind

My wife is a genius at this. I travel a lot. Sometimes she goes with me, but sometimes she doesn't and I'm by myself. I'm around beautiful women all the time but it doesn't matter because Christy has learned to capture my mind. The other day I was traveling and found a card in my suitcase. Cool. We all love surprises. Let me read you the front of the card. "Sometimes when I look at you, I wonder how I got so lucky." You know how guys feel about that? It means nothing to a guy. But here's the part where she captured my mind, when I opened that card, right in the middle was a pair of her panties. All day long, I was thinking about *her*. That entire trip all I was thinking about was her. She's not stupid. She knows how this works. She left that little piece of fabric there for me and captured my mind. It doesn't matter who I meet or what comes up throughout the rest of my day, she has all of my mind. I can't wait to see *her* again. Why? I'm a healthy man. Ladies you can cause a man to be deeply in love with you and chase you the rest of your life if you just do those four things. Here's the best part—you also keep him healthy. It may sound tough or like something you may not *want* to do, but how much do each of these first four steps cost? Trust me, I'm much more expensive. You don't want to have to pay me to help you get your man's testosterone back to normal. These steps cost you nothing, just a little understanding and creativity.

#5 Test the Boy

I often get emails and phone calls from women who have tried #1-4 to tell me it didn't work. Well, then #5 is very important. Back to The Wellness Way motto. *"We don't guess…we test!"*

I had a 31-year-old man and his wife come into my office. Over the course of the last three years he had lost his job, gained a lot of weight and has had zero motivation. Most notably, no sexual drive. It had been two years since he'd had sex with his wife. Does that sound like a healthy boy?

His wife looked at me and said, "If I wasn't a Christian woman, I would have left him already. All I have is a room-mate. I don't want a roommate. I want a husband."

I asked him if he had ever had his hormones tested. You can guess what his answer was. No. But do you know what they did have him on? SIX anti-depressants. In our current way of thinking, the thought was he might have a tumor or fire of some kind. They found nothing, and since they weren't going to cut him open, it was time to use the hose. They kept adding another medication. He was finally on six prescribed medications and in a horrible state! I did the obvious and measured his hormones. I sent him to the hospital where he was getting his psychiatric treatments. Take a look at his levels here:

```
ST. MARY'S HOSPITAL MEDICAL CENTER          GREEN BAY, WI              LABORATORY REP
PATIENT:                                          LOC: SMGLPT
M.R. #                        DOB:                AGE: 31Y          SEX: M
ACCT. #:              DOCTOR: FLYNN, PATRICK MICHAEL                    PAGE: 1

    F4098 COLL: 09/20/2013 11:50  REC: 09/20/2013 11:58 PHYS: FLYNN, PATRICK MICHAEL

    TESTOSTERONE                                                          {SV}
                    L 0.0                  [241.0-827.0] ng/dL
        {SV} = TEST PERFORMED AT ST VINCENT HOSPITAL LABORATORY 835 S VAN BUREN ST GREEN BA
             54301
```

Can you see his levels? No? Because they are 0! Zero. I called the hospital to see if they had made a mistake. They had him come back in and checked it four times. Four. It was consistently the same. Zero. We had figured out what triggered his fires and what he needed to rebuild his house. After three months, we ran his blood work:

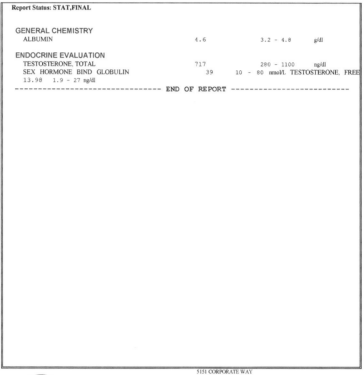

Client: THE WELLNESS WAY 2638 TULIP LN SUITE B GREEN BAY, WI 54313 Phys: FLYNN, PATRICK	11118 Patient: Room# Phone: (920) 429-2844	ID#: Route#:		

:ported on:				
Test Name		**Results**	**Normal Range**	**Units**

Report Status: STAT,FINAL

GENERAL CHEMISTRY
ALBUMIN   4.6   3.2 - 4.8   g/dl

ENDOCRINE EVALUATION
TESTOSTERONE, TOTAL   717   280 - 1100   ng/dl
SEX HORMONE BIND GLOBULIN   39   10 - 80   nmol/L   TESTOSTERONE, FREE
13.98   1.9 - 27 ng/dl
------------------------------ END OF REPORT ------------------------

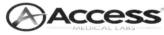

5151 CORPORATE WAY
JUPITER, FL 33458-3101
(866)720-8386

I had them come in to go over his labs, and this time his wife's first words to me were, "Doc, turn it off!"

His body had gone back to normal. We like to see numbers

anywhere over 400 for men's testosterone levels to be in the Man Zone.

Ladies, I have received flack for this next statement, but like I said, I speak it like it is. If your husband is not chasing you every day, he's sick. I don't care if he's 60 or if he's 25. If he's chasing you every day, he's not a pervert or disgusting. He's a real healthy man and you should be thanking God for that.

Guys are easy to understand, easy to get back to normal and easy to keep normal. We have a simple daily and lifelong cycle.

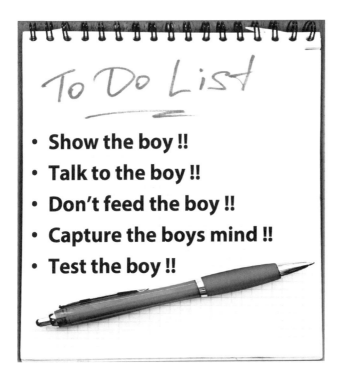

To Do List for Women

Dr. Patrick Flynn

Notes For Myself

_____

_____

_____

_____

_____

_____

_____

_____

_____

_____

_____

_____

Quick Notes For My Partner

_____

_____

_____

_____

_____

_____

_____

_____

_____

_____

_____

_____

_____

_____

Things I'd Like To Discuss With A Wellness Way Doctor

_____

_____

_____

_____

_____

_____

_____

_____

_____

_____

_____

_____

_____

CHAPTER 4

Have you looked ahead to how long this chapter is? Ladies and guys, there's a lot to discuss when it comes to women's hormones. The investment of your time in this chapter will pay off. I'll make this as simple as possible and of course I'll throw in humor.

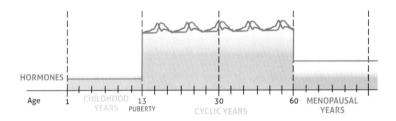

Looks quite a bit different from the graphic we looked at on men's hormones, huh?

Would you agree with me that testosterone causes physical and mental changes? It does, and it is just one hormone. Women have a lot more hormones that change throughout the day, not just throughout the month. Their cycles are very different. Do their cycle and hormones affect them differently than men, both physically and mentally? Of course. How can anybody tell us that men and women are the same? Anyone who politically tells you this is living in a fantasy world. That is why there are so many problems today. Even during counseling, often a man is told to be more sensitive. How's that doing for us right now? Men are not supposed to be overly sensitive. That's not what they are.

One question kept coming back to me and started to become a large piece of my research. Why do women care about everything? Why do they look at everything the way they do? Let's take a day in the life of a woman. From the time a woman gets up in the morning she is the primary person to get the kids ready for school. Have you ever seen a guy dress kids? My wife always asks me how I could let them leave the house dressed like that. They have clothes on. Done. Moms make breakfast, pack lunches, ready the kids for school and then drop them off. They then drive to work where they pour themselves into a multitude of tasks all day. Then they come home and take care of the kids and have to make food again, help with homework and after they've cared for everything all day long-they are exhausted. But this intense schedule means so much to her because it's what she does. She cares. About *everything!*

Now, her man left this morning and he cared about what? *Nothing!* He's got his "one thing" on his mind and is aggressively moving through the day. What is that guy thinking when he comes home? (Insert sexy music here).

And how does the woman respond? "Just another thing I *have* to do!" Ladies, I'm just repeating what you've told me for 18 years. Guys—just understand, it's a thing. It happens and it's real. They are different from us. It's okay to be a man, but you have to understand women are very different; and it's okay to be a woman. They think differently; they care about everything. We don't. Our testosterone keeps us thinking about one thing. We don't think about ten things the way they do. That whole day means a lot to them. Understand that and you'll understand the woman.

Remember when I started the book? I used the word "vagina." I did that on purpose. Women, have you ever noticed a large population of men are interested in hunting? In Wisconsin, where I'm from, we live in a hunting state, so men and women get this analogy. A guy can go to Cabela's, buy deer urine and spray it all over the trees. He can go fishing and scrape the scales off the fish and rip out the guts. He can kill a deer with either a gun or bow and he can rip out the guts right there in the woods with very few tools. But the minute a woman says she has her cycle, he's grossed out. Ever notice that? I used the word "vagina" because I wanted to get under your skin a little, guys. Now that we have a basic understanding, I promise I won't use the word vagina anymore. Ladies, don't worry, we'll still communicate effectively.

We're going to go back to my analogy, we're going to use the example of a house. For the rest of the book, we'll look at the female cycle through a man's point of view. We're going to call it "the Man Cave." The Man Cave changes on a regular basis. Why? There are physical and mental changes going on. All the time. This is what a cycle looks like for a woman through the course of a month:

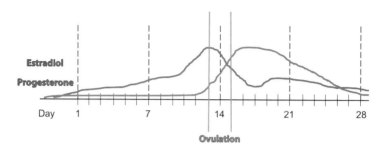

A woman's cycle can range from 26-32 days and it's okay. It can be 27 one time and 29 another. It doesn't have to be the exact same every time. The average cycle for women is about 28 days. Let's look at the hormone patterns. These patterns change on a woman four times a month.

When I got married, my wife looked at me after our pastor said our vows and said, "I do." Guys, this is a very big thing. The pastor should have asked us to say, "I do" four times, because when you say, "I do" to a woman, you 're really marrying four different women. I'm going to show you how this works and it's not as weird as it may sound. Have you ever noticed sometimes your wife can be really awesome and then the following week all you are thinking is "who did I marry?!" You think she's a bit crazy. Guys, you know it's true, but you also have to know that sometimes, crazy is just fine and even okay. Men (and women) don't understand so they think there's something wrong with them when this happens. And when the man tells her she has to be like him, it only makes it worse.

Today's sexual revolution is telling us that women can be as sexually driven as men. No, they can't. If they are as driven as men, they are sick. Let me say it again. If a woman has a sex drive like a man, she is sick and will probably develop cancer someday. Let me explain.

Zone 1: The Construction Zone

This is when the cycle starts. The cycle can go anywhere from 4-7 days. This is when the Man Cave is under construction. I'm being nice here, just think about your woman. Her hormones change, and the first two weeks of her cycle are dominated by estrogens.

Ladies, have you ever heard of the hormone estrogen? Yes? That's why you are sick. There is no such thing. I know, I see the look all the time. It's not "estrogen" it's actually estrogenS. There are multiple estrogens. Estrogens make a lady who she is, just like testosterone makes guys who we are. But let's come back to one thing—if this is what makes each of us who we are, estrogens for women, and testosterone for men—how many of us have had them tested? The method of the fire department is to not worry about anything until your house is on fire. The Wellness Way Approach wants to see normal and keep it that way by preventing fires. Currently the only known cause of breast cancer is a rise in estrogens.

When we test, we are working to keep tabs on those levels and prevent or help our patients recover from the devastation of that horrible disease.

Let's simplify. Let's look at seven estrogens. Yes, I said seven. How many of you have had just seven tested? I'm not talking about all of them, just seven. We wonder why we are so hormonally sick and have so many diseases. Simply stated, those hormones are getting thrown off. However, until you develop cancer, and your house is on fire, the fire department won't show up.

Estrogens are produced by the ovaries. That's important, because later in the month this hormone production will change. What do estrogens do for women? They make them energetic, outgoing, social, enthusiastic, alters their metabolism, and they eat about 15% less than men. It also increases their serotonin—the happy hormone.

Men, pay attention. When the Man Cave is under construction, more oxytocin is released, and her love hormone goes up. Estrogens tell a woman's brain to connect. They don't say "go get it" like your testosterone. Guys you need to learn this. Every guy knows when a woman starts her cycle and the Man Cave is unavailable and he won't be "getting any" he disconnects because he doesn't see the purpose. Again ladies, we are not jerks, just guys. But guys, day one of a cycle is where you can make your wife very sick. Her love hormone has increased and because our sex drive can't be fulfilled, we think we are respecting her by not "pestering." Fair thought. But she needs you and she needs you in a very specific way, maybe just not the way you think. When you separate from her, her love hormone and estrogens drop. We have to understand, it's okay for you to have a sex drive, but this is how *her* body works. When her cycle comes, it's your job to work at connecting with her.

Ladies, if you exercise during The Construction Zone, you run the risk of draining your hormones and pushing your body to be stressed. Your body then thinks it has to produce more hormone. There is one tissue that does a really good job of making hormone. Fat. Yes, the very one you are trying to avoid. If you push your body during the wrong times of the month, during the wrong zones, you can exercise all you want, and you'll gain more fat.

Zone 2: The Man Zone

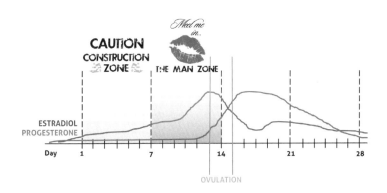

When the cycle stops, and her hormones have come up properly, she enters the zone all of us men are waiting for. She becomes just like you in her sex drive. A woman in her Zone 1 doesn't have much of a sex drive, but as everything increases, so does that sex drive. It's okay and very normal for her sex drive to match her man's at this time. Let's look at those estrogens again. This is the week to exercise. In the Man Zone, it's very important for ladies to exercise. Their bodies can handle it. They also handle stress better, it may even seem like nothing bothers them. Women also burn sugar better in this zone. Have you noticed there are times when you can eat anything and not gain a pound and other times you eat an organic salad and gain five?

Men, here's your chance to help feed her body the right way. We're talking about serotonin, fatty acid, estrogen-based foods. Let's picture a stressed-out woman. Her day was terrible, her husband was a jerk, work was horrible, her kids are driving her nuts and she's craving an organic salad. No. I've never heard a woman say that. When you are stressed, what does your body crave? Chocolate. Do you know why? Chocolate has the highest serotonin content of any food on the planet. Your body knew exactly what it was doing when it sent that craving message.

When I started understanding this, I studied chocolate like crazy. Hershey still sells more chocolate than anyone else in the world. Valentine's Day, February 14, four billion Hershey's kisses are sold. When I'm talking about the health benefits of chocolate, I'm not talking about Hershey or any other over-processed chocolate filled with sugar and chemicals. I'm talking about healthy, real food. There's a very big difference. Don't reach for the bad stuff. That isn't the message your body is sending!

Men, here's a valuable lesson. You can thank me later. There are so many different forms of chocolate. There's cacao beans, nibs, powder, paste, but let me tell you about a little gem called cacao butter. You should feel my hands. They're pretty nice for a guy's hands. Let me tell you why. I'll take some cacao butter and coconut oil and when my wife gets her cycle I'll start rubbing her down and massaging her. Why?

Because I'm a nice guy? No. I'm not a nice guy. I'm no different than you guys. But I understand this so I'm trying to make sure that while she's under the Construction Zone, I'm going to do everything I can to get her into the Man Zone and keep her in the Man Zone. I rub her down and feed her body by rubbing healthy oils and fats on her skin. My hands are so nice because I understand it's my role as her husband to help her through Zone 1 so we can get to Zone 2 and make sure Zone 2 is as good as it can be. Guys, we do have it easy. We keep our testosterone good and things are really simple for us. It's very difficult for a woman. Their bodies change four times in a month. FOUR! I keep saying it, and I will until every man and woman realizes this is normal, not crazy.

With The Wellness Way Approach and our testing, we can help you figure out what specifically each woman needs. We want your husbands to understand this as well because as your body is going through that transition, he should help you with this.

Real life story time. All of these crazy things happen. I've been working with women for a long time. Women will send me the weirdest things. I had a woman one time who was dealing with endometriosis and she had some very large clots during her cycle. Ladies, you know what I'm talking about. One day she came into my office just after she had started her cycle, and she put a baggie containing a baseball-size clot on my desk. She asked me what I thought about that. I told her I didn't think it belonged on my desk. I understood, and she trusted me because I deal with this all the time.

I had a woman come in who was dealing with what I'll call "Man Cave Dryness," I'll let that sink in for a moment (ladies, you know what I mean). She sent me an email after I figured out what her body needed, and she started taking steps to correct her situation. Here's the email:

Dr. Patrick, I wanted to update you and thank you for the advice you gave my husband and me at our last appointment. When you told me the benefits of coconut oil and cacao butter, and how it affects the vaginal tissue I thought you were a little bit crazy. But you've given me good advice so far, so we decided to try it. After applying it vaginally for a couple of days, we started to notice that the soreness started to go down, so we decided to try it out. After a couple of weeks, I'm happy to tell you that I'm starting to enjoy sex again and my husband is very pleased. Not just because we've had more sex in the last couple of weeks than we've had in the last year, but my husband and I have been able to get into positions that I have not been in for over 30 years. He thanks you! Your advice has helped me physically, mentally and brought me closer to my husband.

She's 83.

Alright guys, here's the first of your two *To Do Lists:*

#1 Feed the Girl

Imagine your wife wearing a shirt that says: Feed me chocolate and tell me I'm pretty.

Ladies, if you fast, you'll be very sick. Feed the hormones. For a guy you need to starve their hormones, just one more way we are very different. That's why women can eat hardly anything and still be overweight.

Men, in the first two weeks of their cycle, help them with this. Feed them. They need it. Our thinking is so messed up. If you put fuel in the car and it runs, are you surprised? The car needs gas to run. People are blown away because we do the most simple and basic things and their bodies are changing like crazy. During the first two weeks of her cycle, a woman needs to be eating foods high in fatty acids.

Chocolate-the good kind!
Chia seeds
Pumpkin seeds
Sunflower seeds
Coconut products
Walnuts
Pecans and most other nuts
Olive oil
Hemp
Dates
Avocados
Cherries
Grapes (organic wine is okay)
Maca
Some essential oils that may also help: thyme, lemon and patchouli.

#2 Talk to the Girl

Now that the ladies have read the first part of the book, the guys are loving life because their ladies are taking care of them and understand how their guys work. If guys are confused, they may walk up to their ladies in the morning (because they think their lady is just like them) and say "honey, tonight is going to be a good night!" Guess what is going to happen. Your wife is *NOT* going to come home that night. Why? That doesn't connect with a woman. Don't speak to a woman that way. Treat a lady like a lady. We see the idea of "guy phrases" in movies and while guys think it's great, girls think it's stupid. They know that's not how it works. That doesn't appeal to a woman. Women need connecting words.

There are three words that appeal to a woman. Guys may think it doesn't matter, because she knows it already, but ask my wife. I tell her this all the time. I text her this phrase early in the morning and I'll text it to her in the afternoon. What are the three most important words you can say to a woman?

It's not "I love you."

It's "I choose you." That is one of the most connecting things you can say to a woman. When you disconnect from her, she feels left alone. When she feels disconnected, she'll create things in her head. When you disconnect with her, she thinks you're connecting with someone else. She really does. And she'll play it over in her head and she'll create scenarios and the weirdest things you will ever hear in your life. Most of us have been through it.

About six months ago as I was getting ready to speak to a group, my wife sent me a text message. I thought that was odd, she doesn't send me a text when she knows I'm getting ready to go on stage. But this was special. My 13-year-old daughter was at her first dance at her Christian school. All the girls were standing, swaying back and forth in their pretty dresses. What do you think they were all thinking? *"Come, choose me."* To women this is sweet and precious. Then two minutes later she sent me a picture with this cute 13-year-old blonde boy dancing with my daughter. It meant so much to my wife. Every woman, my wife included, knows how important it is to feel chosen. All I could think is, *"where's my gun?"* I know what those pubescent boys are like. He's no different than any other boy hormonally. Every woman loves to be pursued, to know that she is the focus of her man's affection. It's in their biology. Guys, when you don't chase them, they start to feel disconnected from you.

I've made an observation. Watch out for your friends, ladies. When one of them goes through a divorce or another stressful time, no matter the age, they get very sick quickly. They just do. When a woman feels disconnected and goes through a bad relationship, her hormones drop. Ladies, here's a tip. When your friend is going through a lot of stress, sometimes women can pick up the slack where men are not. That's sad, isn't it? Your friends can help you out just by being a connecting friend. Guys, you can't help each other out that way. Our testosterone won't be driven up by connecting to another man. We're useless with guys.

#3 Touch the Girl

I have gotten thousands of emails on this one.

Guys, *the light switches for the Man Cave are not inside the Man Cave.* I'm going to let that sink in for you guys.

A woman changes four times a month. Finding the light switches can be an adventure. They move every week. It's like looking for Waldo every week. You know this, because you think "I've got this. It was a good night. I touched her there and she loved it." Next week you go to touch her there and she's all: "DON'T touch me!" She's not crazy. Her body changed. One area that was sensitive and felt good one week doesn't feel as good the following week. Guys, when they touch us, it feels good *all the time.* Right? Just make it a game and try to find those light switches. I've had emails that have said it's changed people's marriages, just knowing they each like to be touched differently. She's not him and when he gets that, they're both good.

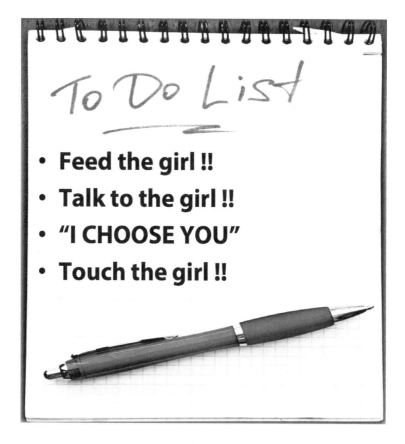

To Do List for Men – Part 1

Zone 3: The Woman Zone

In the middle of her cycle, you have a totally different woman in your house. She flips. Her hormones are totally different. Ladies, hear this clearly, you are normal. You ladies will come to me because your emotions change, and you feel bad. Why would you feel bad? Just like your husband has no control over his morning erection, you have no control over your hormones and emotions changing. None. That should give you ladies a lot of mental peace. You are not supposed to have your emotions flat lined. It's okay for you to go up and down. There's nothing wrong with that. Look what happens in Zone 3:

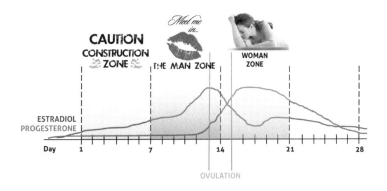

Be very careful guys, you don't know who you are coming home to during this zone. I mean this sincerely, she may bite you. She's normal. Don't make her feel bad because she's emotional and her body is more sensitive to these changes.

With the switch of the hormones, her adrenals take over instead of the ovaries we talked about the first half of the cycle. These are the stress glands. If your body hasn't been adjusted, has chemical stress, and physical stress and you are emotionally stressed out, this week right here will make you very sick. If you exercise too hard during this week, it will make you sick. Your body needs to relax. If you start to stress out, your body will go into the stress response and stress reduces your progesterone. Have you heard of the hormone progesterone? Yes, it's just one hormone. I'm not trying to trick you here. The main job of progesterone is to balance what estrogen does. Progesterone is a calming hormone, and stress can drain it. Progesterone takes estrogens and balances them, so they don't become a problem. Remember how we said if estrogens get too high, you can develop breast cancer?

Let's look at a 70-year-old patient. This woman had gone to her medical doctor and by the time she had gotten to us she was only taking two anti-depressants. She wanted to get off them because she felt she was getting worse. Her son, who is in his 50's, brought her into our office. We had changed his life and he knew we could help her. She had gone through all the tests and exams her general practitioner would have her do and since they hadn't found anything, they put her on a psychiatric drug. I asked her if had they ever tested her hormones. The answer was no.

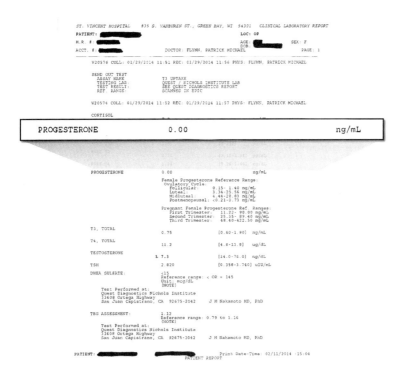

I started with the proper testing. Her progesterone levels were at zero. She sat with me and her son and as we were going over her tests and she started crying. She said three words, "I'm not crazy." Don't confuse hormonal problems with psychiatric problems. There's a combination going on. It's not a separate issue. She's 70, let's look at the other end of the spectrum.

Before I tell this story, I'll tell you this is going to offend many women. I have four daughters, and I have to deal with this personally. Be very careful letting your young daughters play sports. That statement will upset a lot of people. Your little girl isn't the same as a little boy. One good way of building testosterone is moving. Physical exercise can drain a woman's hormones very quickly.

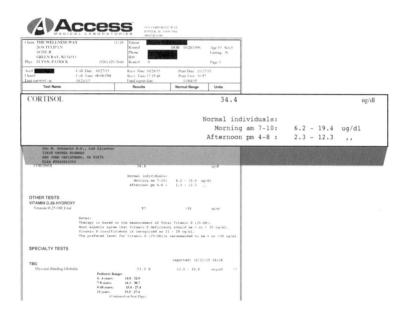

This 19-year-old woman is a runner and a Division 1 scholarship winner for track and field. Do you know what happens to women runners' cycles? They lose them. It's common, but common does not mean normal. The school told her if she didn't run, they'd pull her scholarship. So, as a result, she's physically stressed and mentally stressed and lost her cycle. Why? When you rev the engine really high and don't know how to fuel it, you're going to lose your normal physiology. We tested her stress hormone. It was so high, it was double off the chart even at the lowest value. Yes, you can test stress hormone. It's called cortisol. Remember, hormones are high in the morning and lower at night. If the levels are very high all the time, it's chronic stress. If the levels go very low and they empty out, you experience fatigue. What's the second most common diagnosis given to women today? Chronic Fatigue Syndrome. Let me guess how many of you have had your cortisol tested. Your stress hormones can actually tell your doctor where your body is functioning; high stress or fatigue? Remember The Wellness Way motto? "*We don't guess…we test!*" The whole key is this, we don't test for fires, we test for function. It's very important to get your stress hormones tested, especially if you are a woman. How we take care of you differs as those hormones fluctuate.

Some women tell me they are more of a night person than a morning person. That's why you are sick. Hormones are supposed to be highest in the morning. If you have a hard time getting through the morning and at night when you are not supposed to have much hormone, you feel you can take on the world, your rhythms are off. You are supposed to rest at night. Most people have too much hormone at night and not enough during the day. That's why we ask patients if they are night people or morning people. Their hormones aren't getting high enough at the proper times and that's why they struggle to get their bodies out of bed. At night when you don't need as much, every little bit feels like enough to keep powering through. Now this is a tough one, because most women say they feel fine. They report having a hard time getting out of bed and better able to get a lot done at night. They don't want us to mess up that energy! I understand that, but health needs to come first.

Where do all steroid hormone come from, whether they are male, female or stress hormones? Cholesterol.

I can hear the argument now, "My doctor told me cholesterol is bad for me." If your doctor tells you cholesterol is bad for you, I think he's an idiot. Testosterone comes from cholesterol. Statin drugs became popular in 1984 and are now at an all-time high to reduce cholesterol. How are we doing for heart disease? If a guy is taking a statin drug and his testosterone goes down, what are some of the side effects of the medication? Impotence, heart disease (the very thing it is supposed to help with), loss of motivation, weight gain. That's all on the drug packet insert. Then, we have male enhancement drugs. Let's think about that. They created the problem with one drug. Now they've created another drug to solve the problem created by the first drug. That's crazy! Women weren't often given statins at first but now the number of women on statins is rising rapidly and just about equal with men.

If all of these changes happen as the month goes on, and it doesn't go right, that last zone can be unknown. You don't know who you are walking into that day. But if you take the advice I give you, get tested properly, and help that woman through her cycle, you'll enter the Bonus Zone. She becomes just like you again. If not, it's back to the Woman Zone. How's that for motivation to help your wife out?

Zone 4: The Bonus Zone

Ladies, let me give you a little mental peace. Honestly, you should only have a sex drive about two weeks of the month. Let me say that again. Physiologically you should only have a sex drive two weeks of the month. If you have a sex drive all month long, you are sick and better get checked out. Your husband will be happy, but your hormones have become very abnormal and you're going to end up with some health conditions.

This is the week that will let you know how you did the first three weeks of the month. We either have another Man Zone or another Woman Zone. I think we can all agree which we'd prefer.

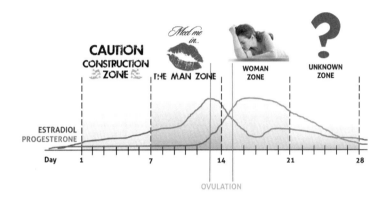

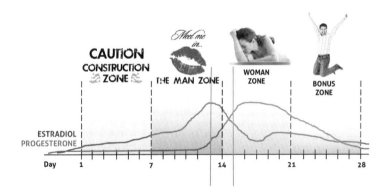

Ok guys, here's your second *To Do List*.

#1 Help the Girl.

I don't just believe this, I know this. It's very difficult to have a woman's body. They change every week. They don't always understand this, so they think there is something wrong with them. Ladies, there's nothing wrong, it's what your body does. Help her to know she is not crazy, she is normal. Help her deal with stress and life. Help her make wise food choices. Help her.

#2 Don't Stress the Girl.

You can be the greatest thing to help her be healthy, or the biggest factor in making her sick. Don't be that kind of guy. It's really sad, but guys don't understand this, and neither do women. Let me give you an example of a situation I had in San Francisco. I was speaking and a woman who considered herself a feminist came up to me and said "Doctor, I disagree. I can handle just as much stress as a man." I asked her why she was there. She said, "because I'm sick." I told her, "take a seat, I think you may learn something." I wasn't being disrespectful, but don't tell me what your body is like and how it functions based on your politics. You don't have to believe me, go home and read it. Mental stress will drain your hormones. Physical stress will drain your hormones. Chemicals will drain your hormones. Guys, are lucky in that stress does not affect our hormones. The guy can have a horrible day. Work was challenging, the kids' behavior sucked, and still he gets home at night and what does he want? SEX. A lady has stress, and guys, you know those panties are pretty much super glued on. Right? Why? It changes their body when they stress out. Ladies, you may not want to hear this, but you can't handle stress like a man, you never will, and your biology will never let you. Men, it's your job to reduce the stress of a woman. This alone should relieve stress for women.

#3 Protect the Girl

I got home one day, and I could tell right away that my wife and daughter were not having a good time. Christy told me, "Go talk to your daughter!"

So, I took Faith to our favorite organic tea spot and after a little chatting she starts "Daddy…"

I interrupted her, "whoa, whoa, whoa, before you say anything, remember this, that's my wife. I will protect my wife from anybody, including you. So, when you go home, you're going to go and apologize to your mother. Remember, if you make her stressed out, you can make her sick. You are eventually going to leave her, I'm not."

After a while, we went home, and they talked. I still to this day don't even know what the problem was. The next morning when I went to wake Faith, she said "Daddy, before you go, I just want to say I'm sorry for making Mom mad last night."

I told her, "Don't worry, God forgives, just move on."

She went on to say, "Daddy, I've been thinking about it a lot. I know why I drive Mom so crazy."

"Really, you do?"

"Yeah, I'm just like you!" Where did she come up with that?! Christy would tell you she's the image of me in every way. When men get stressed, they'll leave their wife and bond to their kids. Don't do that. Bond to your wife. She needs you two to stay connected. Protect her, even from her own kids.

#4 Schedule with the Girl

The greatest thing a guy could say to his wife in the morning would be "honey, would you like to go on a date with me?" Oh guys, if you could only see the room full of smiling ladies I see when I say this in one of my seminars. Guys, when you first met that woman, you did everything. Your testosterone was driven, you created pictures in your mind and you chased her and you dated her, and you scheduled things with her. She's still the same way, but most guys have stopped doing those things. Her biology will always desire to connect with you. One of the best things guys can do is to continue to date their wives. If you do this, and you plan it, she'll create the picture in her mind of all the wonderful things that make you to be the most amazing man in her world. Guys, how much does that cost you? It pays off huge. Plan it. You plan it, guys. When you were first chasing her and pursuing her, you planned everything. Then when you married her, it became "what do you want to do?" Don't do that. You plan it, that connects with her. Take her somewhere peaceful to sit and just ask her "honey, how was your day?" That gives a woman the opportunity to talk for the next three and a half hours and you don't have to do anything. When she talks, she's connecting. What does that do to her hormones? It makes her healthy. Think about that. It's very simple.

Now I hear, "Doc, we do all of these things and my wife still doesn't respond."

#5 Test the Girl

Today, women deal with more hormonal problems than ever in history and they are as sick as can be. It's why we have more fertility problems and more cancers.

This concept we started 18 years ago has become a national brand for this reason. It's a different thought process that's easy to apply with a doctor that does things right. When we apply this different process to patients, we get different results. What are we getting from medicine? Right now, based on medical statistics, 1 out of 2 of you would die of heart disease. 1 out of 3 would die of cancer. If you don't change your thinking, you're going to end up like them. Remember, don't accept common for normal.

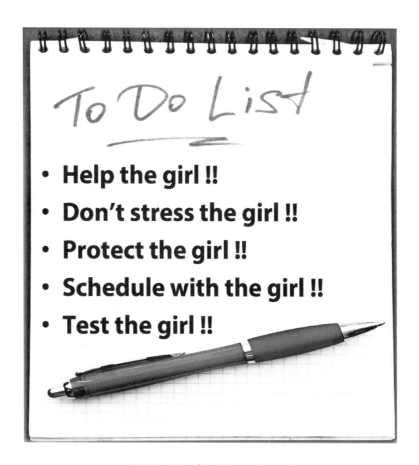

To Do List for Men – Part 2

Notes For Myself

_____

_____

_____

_____

_____

_____

_____

_____

_____

_____

_____

_____

_____

Quick Notes For My Partner

_____

_____

_____

_____

_____

_____

_____

_____

_____

_____

_____

_____

_____

Things I'd Like To Discuss With A Wellness Way Doctor

_____

_____

_____

_____

_____

_____

_____

_____

_____

_____

_____

_____

_____

CHAPTER 5

Menopause is a bad word for many women. Women do not have to experience the difficult "symptoms" of menopause that cause most women to cringe and fear the experience even before they enter this natural process. There aren't many women throwing parties for this transition in their life. First, let's understand what menopause is and what it isn't.

When you say the word menopause to a woman, do they think "healthy, vital and sexual" right away? No. They think vaginal dryness, period problems, night sweats. That's not menopause. If you have any of these problems, that's a sign that you are sick. Menopause doesn't have to be that way.

Standard medical thinking and approach treats menopause like a disease; like an angry monster that when you hit 50 years old will reach around your bed and grab you.

While this is a natural transition, it's very different from anything a man experiences. For a guy, we hit puberty and then we die. That's about it; if we keep ourselves healthy.

The largest medical establishment in the country is Mayo Clinic. Mayo defines menopause perfectly, well, the first part of their definition anyway. They define it perfectly, then they mess it up in my opinion.

Yes, Mayo Clinic has it all wrong.

Menopause is defined as occurring 12 months after your last menstrual period and marks the end of the menstrual cycles. Menopause can happen in your 40s or 50s with the average American woman beginning at age 51.

Ladies, if you go through menopause in your 40s, that's alright, just get your hormone levels tested to be sure that is what is really happening.

Menopause is a natural biological process. Although it also ends fertility, you can stay healthy, vital and sexual. Some women feel relieved because they no longer worry about pregnancy.

Right there, everything Mayo Clinic said to that point is perfect. They should have stopped. Our current system can teach women about menopause to a point but then it takes on a negative connotation. If I were to walk up to a woman and tell her "menopause keeps you healthy, vital and sexual" they'd look at me and ask, "what planet are you from?"

Moving onto Mayo's next paragraph, after that perfect definition, they totally lose their credibility and confuse women.

Even so, the physical symptoms such as hot flashes, and emotional symptoms of menopause may disrupt your sleep, lower energy and for some women trigger anxiety and feelings of sadness and loss.

It can't be both. How can you be healthy, vital and sexual with that list of symptoms? Let me make this clear. Menopause is a natural biological state and process. Recently, Mayo updated their definition, I wonder if we had an impact on that.

I had a woman come in to see me. Her primary complaint was how she was suffering so badly from menopause symptoms. She was 64. Guess what my first question was. Have you ever had your hormones tested? I wanted her to say it out loud, so she could hear it herself. You already know her answer. Nope. I tested her hormones and they were devastatingly bad. We had discovered what was causing the fire and built her hormones back to their proper levels and retested.

The next time I saw her our conversation went like this, "Doc, I'm doing so awesome, I feel amazing. I feel healthy, vital, and sexual!"

To which I replied, "Thank goodness I got rid of your menopause!"

She looked at me like I had grown a second head. I knew right away she had caught what I had said. I didn't get rid of her menopause! Menopause is a state of life if you live long enough. The only way for a woman to avoid it is to die young.

Because it's so common for women to have this long list of symptoms during menopause: irregular periods, hot flashes, vaginal dryness, night sweats, mood changes, weight gain, thinning hair, breast fullness, they believe those symptoms *are* menopause. This is not menopause. This means you are sick. Your hormone levels are off. Just because these are so common, women have accepted it as normal. Don't confuse common with normal. Is PMS normal? Why is it a "syndrome?" Your doctor accepts it as normal and teaches women to do the same.

When The Wellness Way doctors come along and talk about hormones and the basic biology of this transition; all of a sudden it makes sense. It doesn't matter which Wellness Way Clinic across the country you go to or which doctor you see there, we all look at it from the same perspective. The body doesn't make mistakes. If women go through those symptoms, it's a signal their bodies are struggling as they are going through the change.

Our testing approach is different. We get a complete picture of what is going on and start to find out what is throwing those hormones off so that we can help women live in that healthy, vital, sexual state of menopause.

The only thing medicine can do is create some sort of synthetic hormone for women that will cause cancer. They've set women up for this devastation and decline in health. Women don't have to go through all these physical and psychological challenges. Yes, the synthetic hormone works to relieve the symptoms, but the side effect is cancer. That's not a fair trade.

When women are suffering with menopause, men can't be sympathetic because a man can hardly detect a slight change in his own hormones. A woman's hormones are so physically connected to her body from her big toe to her brain. When that transition is off, it will cause a woman emotional disruption, as well as physical disruptions including her sleep. We all know how that will end. That's not menopause. You are sick.

I'm sure some jaws will drop here, but I wish menopause for my wife. We have our four beautiful babies, and we've decided not to have anymore. I wish my wife could just go through menopause so she wouldn't have to deal with her cycle anymore. Does that sound like something any other man would wish for his wife if menopause is truly a horrible event? It is so much easier to keep a woman's hormones healthy and normal when she isn't cycling. A menopausal woman's hormone cycle isn't any different than a guy's really, it's just a flatline that's easy to keep right where it should be.

I had the blessing of helping my mom through this transition. Many people ask me what I did to help her. Well, first they ask me if I like taking care of my mom, especially through menopause. Yes. There's nobody better to do this than me! I want my mom to be healthy. I did run specific tests on her based on what I knew about her. There are multiple test options; blood, saliva, and urine. It depends on the woman and her situation. Each woman is unique and needs to be approached as such, not as a standard procedure. Based on her results there were many options to help her, but I needed to know how to focus on *her*.

The first step is changing the way you think about menopause and the way you approach your health care. If you took one of the test results I ran to a medical doctor, he'd look at the test from the perspective of which medication he is going to put you on. We are going to rebuild your house so you aren't dependent on a synthetic hormone or worse yet, a psychiatric drug for the rest of your life. You can not only survive menopause but thrive and live a life that is healthy, vital and sexual. Your body was created to go through menopause as a healthy stage of life.

Things I'd Like To Discuss With A Wellness Way Doctor

_____

_____

_____

_____

_____

_____

_____

_____

_____

_____

_____

_____

_____

CHAPTER 6

Each week I do a live recording of *"The Dr. Patrick Flynn Show."* Viewers and patients send us questions, so we can respond live and unscripted. It's a great outlet for so many questions to be answered while getting the right information to people seeking answers. Here's a question and my response from one episode.

Hi Dr. Patrick, I am 32 years old and we have 3 children. My husband does not want anymore but I would not mind; because of that he wants me on birth control. I started taking it and I don't feel good; I don't even feel like the same person! I've gained weight, I'm more emotional, but my husband said he will NOT use condoms. I've been following you for a long time and know it's not good for me and the more I research I do, I'm scared that I'm taking it. What research can I give him to convince him that I should not be on it? Also, he says it is fine because my OB said it was the best way to prevent another pregnancy.

This is one of those areas I will probably answer differently than you would expect. First, we'll take this from the relationship side.

Ladies, this is an interesting situation. Women will take care of their bodies. However, the minute their husband wants them to do something different, they will in a heartbeat. Typically, this is due to the deep need for connection and to keep the peace in the relationship they desire. You want research? Stop having sex with him. There's your research. Unless he uses condoms, you aren't having sex. Ladies, understand, you have the control.

I know I'll hear from Christian ladies out there, "But Doc, being a Christian woman, I just have to do what he wants and submit." My friend Ross Allen Skorzewski, who is my host on "*The Dr. Patrick Flynn Show,*" has worked in the church for over 20 years and has plenty of experience in marriage and relationship counseling. He has also worked with one of the greatest marriage enrichments speakers in the world, Pastor Mark Gungor. Here's his response to this argument:

Stop over-spiritualizing this situation. If he is putting you in an unhealthy place, and now we are talking about birth control, you need to look at this more clearly. He says he won't use condoms. The only option for him to be intimate with you is for you to put this unhealthy poison into your body. You need to rattle that boy's cage. You need to get a hold of him and shut down the shop and say, "The Man Cave is closed." This isn't about submitting, this is about dysfunction junction. He needs to look at his relationship with his wife and not just his own needs. He may just want sex now, but he'll be getting a lot less of that as his wife's body gets sicker. The dysfunction has to stop. This has to be about a healthy relationship and healthy bodies, together.

According to the email, it doesn't even look like it was a discussion, and often it's not. He may have said he won't use condoms and she needs to take birth control. Because she desires that relationship, she caves. If she would just hold out and be strong, after a short time he'll use condoms. Guess what's going to happen. His testosterone will build up and his sperm retention will go to his brain…ladies, trust me, you have more control over him than you think.

Here's another angle to this, the OB said it was the best thing for her to use to prevent pregnancy. It doesn't mean it's best for *her body*. But there is an even better way to prevent pregnancy. Abstinence. Shut it down. You'll have no kids. You'll frustrate that guy, but you won't have to worry about pregnancy. The moment you tell him no, he'll go for a period of time without being intimate with you, but he'll quickly consider the use of condoms.

Let's look at it from the health standpoint. Birth control is very detrimental to female health. It is an endocrine disrupter as defined by the EPA. It throws off the cycle and trust me, you'll end up with problems. The woman who sent the email did emotionally break down and take the birth control. She knew right away she was starting to feel sick. Picture this. If the average person who has no problem takes a medication it makes them sick. Remember what medication does? It forces a response. Actually, medication by pharmacology definition is a non-lethal dose of a lethal substance. If a healthy person takes a medication they become sick. This woman has three beautiful kids and apparently no problems with pregnancies and now goes on a hormone disrupter. She's going to feel sick.

This woman now doesn't feel like the same vibrant person she was before the birth control. Every time she looks at herself, she's probably bothered by the weight gain and her emotions are completely off. She's not going to *want* to get naked! She's going to shut down because of all the changes going on in her body. Women, you are so subconscious about your bodies. Most guys don't care about the subtle changes like weight gain in your body. But for you, this is huge and will disrupt your whole being. You need to stay strong and say no. If he becomes disrespectful and disruptive, you know what kind of man you are dealing with. You're not his puppet. He doesn't control you, especially in causing you health problems. He is setting her up for both health and relationship failure.

I would hope that men would have their wives' best interest in mind; her health and physiology, her emotions, their relationship and even her husband's health. Because if they did *and* understood what birth control does, they wouldn't ask their ladies to put this into their bodies. This will inadvertently affect him as well, because she won't want to be intimate with him. Or, she'll have sex because she feels obligated. She will have sex because it's the only way to be intimate with her husband. "If I say no, he'll stop loving me." If he becomes a jerk, you need to rattle that boy's cage, because it's obvious that his eyes are more on what he wants than what is best for you and his relationship with you.

Men, if you play this card you are making your wife sick and behaving very selfishly. Get over it.

The wife wants to give him research. He doesn't want research. He's not going to look at it. The OB said it was the best way to avoid pregnancy. He's going to use that leverage. Your doctor would be right in that it is *ONE* of the best ways to avoid pregnancy, but it's also one of the most devastating things to the health of her body. He's taking it out of context. If you really want to hand him something to read, hand him that paper that comes in the pack of pills. Death is an amazing way to avoid pregnancy. But that's not the goal. Here's the research, how are *you* feeling? That's proof enough, or at least it should be.

Ok, so most women and maybe some men want conclusive research. I get it. Take a saliva hormone test before you start a birth control and after you've been taking it a little while. That hormone shows up in your bodily fluids, not just your blood stream. It is also in your saliva and your vaginal secretions. Every time you kiss him, or you have sex with him, he gets the hormone. You are passing it to him. I have men come into the office and their estrogen and progesterone levels are way off. They ask me how it's possible. Is your wife on birth control? Well, then you're taking it too. When he gets that these hormones are also affecting his body and will create problems for him as well, he's quick to get her off that poison.

"Doc, are you telling me to use sex as a weapon or a tool against my husband to get him to follow hook, line and sinker?" Well, at some point you're going to have to do something. A man will respond. You're not getting him to buy you a new car or a new house. You're using this to stand up for your health because you are getting sick.

One of the number one side effects of birth control? Cancer. Remember that insert of info from the pill packet. That will list all the disruptions it will cause in the woman's body, including cancer. He'll get a whole lot less sex if her body and family is devastated by cancer.

Ladies, you need to take care of you. You need to take a stance to take care of your health. He may justify with reasons, but he doesn't live in your body. Don't feel guilty because you are making the best decision for your body. If you get cancer, it could cost you your life and/or your family money as well as resentment. Don't let that seed be planted. It will divide your relationship.

Things I'd Like To Discuss With A Wellness Way Doctor

_____

_____

_____

_____

_____

_____

_____

_____

_____

_____

_____

_____

CHAPTER 7

Recently a question that has come up in the office, from other friends and family and has been featured on my weekly *"The Dr. Patrick Flynn Show"* is about young girls entering puberty and developing at a young age. Here's a question we featured from one of our viewers:

Hi Dr. Patrick. What is with all of the young girls getting boobs so early? My niece is a few years older than my daughter and turns 8 in November. My sister said she is already showing signs of puberty. I thought I had years before I had to worry about that! My mom says it is because of all the hormones in the meat. Is she right? Should I stop feeding my daughter meat? Do I need to worry since this is happening to my niece, will it also happen to my daughter? They are related.

Having daughters, I get extremely serious about this. If you go back in history, even 50 years ago, the average start of menstruation is 15-16 years old. If you look at Biblical times, the Bible is such great documentation of history, most people were married and sometimes having kids right after menstruation began. Could you imagine if your daughter had her cycle at 10 years old? Go back in history and with menstruation starting at 15, 16 or even 17, these young women were almost adults already. What has been the change that has happened to cause early development?

Our genome has not changed. The whole idea of our genetics controlling this aspect is ridiculous, although many in the medical world will play the genetics card. The purpose of genetics is to keep your body normal, to support life. When you are born your genes make sure you develop to a healthy and normal state. If there is disruption during development, you can see some changes. Your life may not be as extensive, but you can still live a very healthy life.

If you come back to what is possibly going on, you have to look at all of the things that could trigger changes to develop that much quicker. The meat and hormone issues are very well known and well documented, but it's just one factor.

They put the hormones into the cow to increase the growth rate and the mass of that animal. If you go back 200-300 years ago, the only people who ate muscle meat were the peasants, the slaves, and people of lower social statuses. Organ meats were the delicacy. The king wouldn't eat a muscle meat, that's peasant meat. But muscle meat can be mass produced and is readily available and frequently consumed. If you talk to a young person about an organ meat, they freak out. Grandma's house had liver paste. We sat there eating heart, liver, kidney, and tongue. The farming industry got people to shift away from organ meats because you can't produce them at a high rate like you can muscle meat. Now instead of grass feeding them, we're grain feeding them which will make them grow even faster. If you notice the highest expense in your meat is not based on its weight, it's based on quality. It's the only industry that we've moved away from quality. Your cars get better every year and the food system gets crappier every year. It's about speed, it's about convenience. That's why as a culture we've allowed our foods to fall to such a terrible quality. I get people who say "Doc, healthy food is so expensive." Do you ever ask the question why crappy food is so cheap? Most of it's not food.

The industry has focused on getting the animal to be larger, to weigh more so they can sell more as quickly as possible. If you ingest those hormones in the meat, you're going to alter your hormones. They are sticking these growth hormones into the meat that are causing women's estrogens to go up higher than they are supposed to and it's inducing faster maturity and puberty. So yes, meat can do it, but it's not the only thing. Let's be clear, I am not saying to quit eating meat. I'm saying get a good source. Ask a local organic farmer what they feed the cow and buy half a cow. It's cheaper and healthier.

There are so many other triggers. Meat is just one. If there is an introduction of hormones into any food source, it can induce early maturation and puberty. Do you know what the number one source for everyone-male, female, and child-to come in contact with hormones? It's not meats. The number one source of hormone introduction to the human body comes from city water.

Not long ago, I went up to see my sister in Spokane, Washington. We went to the gorgeous river. Right next to it was a water treatment facility. They're sucking the water and cleaning it out and pushing it back into the system. When we drove by, I pointed out to my sister that there's no filtration. When a woman who takes birth control pills pees, it goes into the water system and gets recycled back. Filtration is very important. If you do not have proper water filtration on your house, enjoy everyone else's hormones in your showers, your cooking, and your drinking water.

There are so many things considered endocrine disruptors that will also raise the estrogens levels in young girls. Many of them we come into contact with daily. The heavy metals in dental fillings, plastic water bottles and food storage, soft plastic toys and vinyl, metal cans for canned food, household cleaners and fragrances, flame retardants on children's pajamas and other household products all contain endocrine disruptors that change reproductive hormones.

There is one more "healthy food" that needs to be addressed. Soy. Soy contains phytoestrogens. These are plant-based compounds that mimic human hormones. Soy is very prevalent in our processed foods today. It is used in so many ways throughout the food industry that you are still most likely getting soy even when you don't realize it. Then there are the "health" freaks who say they are avoiding meats and turn to soy as a protein source. So, you see, avoiding meat isn't the answer either!

There are multiple things that can drive up estrogens levels. The only thing to cause the change from child to young womanhood is those estrogen levels coming up. If they are forced synthetically, your gene system will respond to the environment and bring on puberty. There is no reversing this effect.

So yes, we are looking at this issue of breasts getting bigger and earlier in girls. The mother was right that the meat source is possibly one of the issues due to the hormones that have been injected into that animal. Change that source of meat, don't eliminate meat altogether. Also, take a look at some of the other exposures to hormones through the diet that may need to be addressed. Does she need to worry because they are related? No, this is not a genetic issue, but if both sets of parents do the same things, the kids could have similar reactions. Your genes respond to help you to live the longest and healthiest life possible. You are not genetically programmed to suffer or be sick.

Things I'd Like To Discuss With A Wellness Way Doctor

CHAPTER 8

Sometimes I have people tell me that the care they get from The Wellness Way is too expensive. I want to share a story with you.

This story is about a woman named Patty, her husband Josh and their heartache in trying to start a family. Eleven years ago, Patty and her husband Josh tried to get pregnant. After trying for eleven years, guess what happened, nothing. She went to the medical doctors. They only have two tools, they gave her medications, did she get pregnant? No. She didn't. So, they only had one tool left, they decided to do IVF therapy. They extracted 3 eggs from her ovaries and fertilized them, then they implanted one. Any guess how much that cost? $20,000. Insurance covers nothing. I apologize guys, but I don't feel sorry for you if you are mad over the cost of real health care. I'm here to get you to change your life so you aren't sick and divorced.

Patty paid the $20,000 and it did not work. They implanted the second egg for $20,000 and that didn't work. The doctors told Patty and her husband that they had one more egg left, and they felt bad for her since she had already spent $40,000 so they'd do the last one for $5,000. But before they did this, the doctors said they'd heard about this guy in Green Bay, Wisconsin. They didn't really know what I do, but they told her, "He gets crazy results."

Patty and her husband came into The Wellness Way. As we were going through her medical records, I asked her some very basic questions. "Did they test your hormones?"

"No."

Well, they actually had tested one of them, but they were incomplete in their testing. So, we did test her hormones accurately and they were off. I started to go through the process to figure out what was going on with her. I started finding the triggers and rebuilt her body. After 9 months we retested her, and she was regaining healthy levels of hormones; I sent her back to her doctor. They did the last in-vitro and she got pregnant. I was so happy for her and Josh.

But here's what medicine does. Medicine has standards they do with everyone. One of the standards they do with IVF is to give the woman hormone shots to keep her pregnant. Since the body generally hasn't been brought to a place of healthy function, they need to manipulate those hormone levels to maintain the pregnancy. Josh, Patty's husband, called me and was concerned they wanted to do these hormone shots. "Doc, is this okay?" I told him, "Her labs are normal; the shots will make her abnormal and make her sick. "

She went back to the doctor and the doctor told her "Dr. Patrick is hurting you, don't go back to him. You have to do this. If you do not, we won't take care of you."

I'm sorry guys, but I think most of your doctors are a bunch of idiots. They say the stupidest things, especially when it comes to me and The Wellness Way Approach. I don't care if that offends you. What have they done? They've poisoned you, they've said things to you that are not true and what has happened? You are sick. I work with infertile women, and those with cancer all the time and people say, "my doctor said this…" I don't care what your doctor said. Your doctor said something I gave you could hurt you. He's an idiot if he thinks anything I do could hurt you. There isn't one thing we can give you that would hurt you. It can't, it doesn't work that way.

So, did Patty listen to them or me? She was scared so she listened to them. Six weeks later, in October, that baby died. The doctor in his arrogance said, "you can't have children" and left. He wouldn't step foot back into the room or answer any questions for her. Not one. She had trusted this doctor, and he turned his back on her.

She went into a deep depression after she lost the baby. Josh texted me and called me often saying, "I can't get Patty out of bed she's so depressed." I told him to leave her be, she had to get her stress down. A month later I hadn't heard from them and then Josh reached out to me again. "Doc, Patty's finally getting up and around. You made the most sense to us even when the doctors said the most horrible things about you. My wife was the happiest and healthiest when she was with you. I understand we can't have a baby, but I'd rather have my wife happy and healthy than sick with no child."

I told him, "I don't care what the doctors said. I think they are idiots. But don't tell your wife that. I'll do what we need to do." Those other doctors had messed her body up so badly with all those hormones. I had to detox her and build her hormones back properly. That detox was painful for her; they put all this junk into her body. She felt like she was going to die. February 8th, I called Patti, so we could redo her labs. She said that she and Josh were going to go on vacation to Mexico for three weeks. I told her to call me when she got back.

March came around and all of a sudden, I got a text message from Patty. She said "Dr. Patrick, I was at work today and my boobs were sore, I was tired, and I got nauseous, so I went to Walgreens and I bought seven pregnancy tests and they are all positive. How did that happen?!"

Recently she sent me a picture of her son, "Joshua wanted to say hi to his favorite doctor!"

Why am I his favorite doctor? Because the other doctors had given up hope and destroyed his parents hopes of having children. Their thinking and philosophy were different than the one Patty and her husband needed. They can tell you that I'm wrong in every way. They can say bull crap like I've hurt you, but I need to ask you, "How healthy are you? Are you in the same position as before? Worse?"

You can tell your doctor I said he is an idiot. I'm sick and tired of people being sick, infertile, unhappy, and divorced. I'm done being nice. I will start being nice when cancer, heart disease and all common diseases start decreasing. Until then I hope I offend everyone. If I am not doing the right thing, why is The Wellness Way a national brand? Why are people calling us from all over the world to come speak to their audiences? This concept can be implemented by so many doctors across the world to make a difference in people's lives. The doctors who come to us, to be a part of what we do, have good hearts and just want to take care of people.

I will continue to do this, even with the death threats, the hate mail and all the nasty things said about us. We will continue to do the right thing. We challenge you to do the right thing for your health.

PATIENT TESTIMONIALS

A note from Christy

On being the first patient of The Hormone Whisperer:

I'm just a small-town country girl who fell in love with an amazing small-town guy. He had a vision in his heart to help people regain their health. I'm honored to have been his first patient in this way and to see where it has led. It's overwhelming to think I had some small part in that.

I remember the day Patrick came to my place and I was on the floor in a fetal position. There were a lot of emotions. I remember him just brushing it off when I told him I was probably not going to be able to have children. He said, "I disagree, don't worry." I figured we would cross that bridge when we got there. He was so sure, and I trusted in that.

Patrick was the only person willing to connect the dots for me. He was the only person who bothered to look for a solution. He gave me hope. I had learned enough to know I wanted to do things naturally. I was already under chiropractic care, but what I didn't know was the power of chiropractic care. Many people only think of chiropractic care as pain management for physical trauma. There is a whole philosophy of chiropractic relating to the 3T's (thoughts, toxins and trauma) unknown to so many people. Once I understood what true health came from, there was no turning back. I met Patrick and I never stepped foot into another OB/GYN's office. That was it. I was all-in. I never looked back. He practiced adjusting on me. He took me to all his chiropractor friends who had graduated before him, I was adjusted by all of them including doctors with whom he had interned. Patrick was determined to figure out why my body was so sick and to return it to normal.

We did some dramatic things such as eliminating sugar completely from our lives! I remember the day like it was yesterday. I cried. I was emotionally addicted. My mother and grandmother had taught me to bake. It was how we showed love and care for our family. I had to make a decision; to be healthy or remain sick. Now, years later, I love to create new recipes using healthier ingredients comparable to those treats from long ago in the kitchens of my childhood. It's not easy. You have to make a choice. Treat everything you put into your mouth as either bringing life or bringing death.

Patrick proposed to me outside of a new hospital. I imagine this may not sound like the traditional engagement story, but it is a huge part of our story. We were walking the quiet path on the hospital grounds with the soft lights and large snowflakes falling around us. I didn't truly understand at that point. Can anyone really understand what is to come? It was romantic in *our* way. I understood his heart, his dreams and vision. I knew as long as we would walk through it together, it would be worth it. He was proposing to the woman he loved in front of the paradigm and dogma he battled. He told me if I agreed to be with him for the rest of our lives, it would include a journey-an uphill battle. Patrick wanted me to know I was saying yes to not only him, but this life. I knew no matter how hard it would get or what the adversities we faced, it would all be worth it.

When he proposed to me, did I have any inkling that our life would look anything like it does? No! Oh, my goodness, no! When I was a kid and dreamed of my life, I would never dream past age 25. I would never dream about marriage or life past that point. Ironic, we got married when I was 25 and my life completely changed. I couldn't have pictured it if I had tried.

In the beginning this new life was a struggle. I lived on an island for many years, going against the grain. No one was doing what we were doing. As the years went by we built a community of people, educating and inspiring them to become healthier and to create healthy families. We created the community we needed right in Green Bay, Wisconsin. The dynamics of our city changed. We had patients go to the grocery store requesting healthier ingredients eliminating the need to have to drive to Milwaukee on a regular basis just to stock our pantries. This community of people who used to be sick and unhealthy became a transforming group of like-minded individuals. They were taking a stand for what was needed for their own health and their families.

When we were ready to start our family with children and stopped trying to "not get pregnant", I got pregnant right away. I was so excited. We told people right away. We didn't live in fear. We didn't seek the hospital route. Instead, we chose to have our sweet and precious babies at home with a midwife.

Don't allow someone to tell you it's not possible. Don't allow someone to try to scare you or make you believe lies. God created us to be mothers. We need to support and encourage each other. We need to reinforce this within a broken healthcare paradigm. There is a different way-The Wellness Way. This is the pathway to create a healthy family. We need to ask a different question to find the answers we need. What isn't functioning correctly? Why isn't it functioning correctly? Be willing to approach hurdles in a different way than you have before. You may be amazed at the people who come across your path who have the answers to the prayers you've prayed.

I'm excited for the many people who can be helped by The Wellness Way. This is about getting results. The principles and testing allow us to give people hope, answers, and the ability to see things differently. Patrick always talks about the importance of being able to step back and approach your challenges with a different mindset. The Wellness Way approach is an idea – an idea that says we are not genetically programmed for disease or illness, but for health. It's based on the philosophy that you can only truly be healthy if you address all 3T's. We test because everyone is unique and should be treated that way. How are these 3T's affecting you specifically? The Wellness Way focuses on who you are and what you need; not a standard procedure.

This book and seminar help people look at all healthcare options. If we could do that for one person, it has all been worth it. The best part is in knowing so many people can be helped. After Patrick started helping me, women began coming from all over. They included a friend my age who was prescribed pre-menopausal drugs, to others who were given no choice but to take some form of artificial hormone. Word travels fast. We now have women calling The Wellness Way from all over the world. I've been able to watch as Patrick has been able to offer different answers to so many women. He's given hope to those who want to bear children, building their own legacy and future family, while impacting their children's children. Raising those healthy kids is another whole adventure! We are creating a healthier society, one baby and momma at a time.

Looking forward, I'm excited to create a different legacy of thought. I don't fear my girls not having babies. I'm excited. I talk to our girls about having children and a large family if they choose. It is joyous to discuss bringing life into the world and doing what God has called us to do as women. He's given us gifts to do what men cannot. The gift to be mothers. I want my girls to embrace it. To know that being a mother is a blessing. A gift. It's something to be celebrated and not treated as if it were a disease to be fixed or medicated.

I'm very proud of the man Patrick has become and I'm excited to see how God continues to use him. I'm blessed to be on this journey with him and I can't imagine life without him. He's affected so many people and I'm inspired by that man's brain, but most of all his heart. Of course, he's good looking, but ultimately, talking with him; the way his brain works is so intriguing. I could listen to him teach all day. I wanted to marry an intelligent and intriguing man. I love learning from him and how we look at the future-learning, growing and continuing on this journey together. My husband is the most generous, honest, and caring man. He never stops researching. He seeks out the best quality labs and products to ensure the greatest results in all the clinics across the country. The only variable is what *you* will choose.

On the To Do Lists:

As he was coming up with the *To Do Lists*, Patrick started telling me about the things I was doing to help our marriage. I wasn't even aware that I was following a *To Do List*! Every once in a while, I'll gauge myself to make sure I'm keeping up with my end of the *To Do Lists*. Even though I helped to create them, I know I need to stay mindful to continue with them for our marriage. They can change a marriage. I know what marriage is like before the *To Do Lists* and the results once they are implemented. Every marriage has struggles but having useful tools helps point the way to a better marriage. Use the tools and the *To Do Lists*. Both the husband and the wife need to come to a point where they are humble enough to recognize the needs of the other person need to come first and be met. We need to recognize we don't have to be the same. Patrick and I are two totally different people. When you respect and recognize each other's differences, celebrate and embrace them, an amazing marriage can be built. When women complain and nag, I just want to pull them aside and tell them they don't understand their husband. Likewise, a husband shouldn't be stressing his wife. He may not under-stand that he is causing her to stress and in doing so depleting her hormones. It's a two-way street. If a husband and a wife can humble themselves and honestly look at what they need to change in their own behaviors and actions, it's a recipe for a better relationship.

Ladies, I encourage you, your partner may not want to

read the book (his hormones may not let him sit still that long). He *will* love the seminar. He will enjoy the entertaining approach. You'll leave with real tools to put to work right away. Get you *and your husband* to a seminar. Almost every woman who comes to the seminar without her husband tells us, "I wish I would have brought my husband!" If you are looking for answers or highly entertaining information, you'll find it at The Hormone Connection seminar. It's a fresh perspective and look at a topic that affects every man, woman and family. Check in with your nearest Wellness Way clinic for The Hormone Connection seminar schedule. It will change your life.

When a partner can gain insight into their marriage and what could be going on physiologically, hopelessness is born into new hope. This isn't just a story. This is the dedication and passion of our life. This is our real-life story. I believe it gives hope.

This man is the love of my life. He's the incredible father of our four beautiful girls. From daily dance parties when daddy gets home each night, to watching an occasional romantic "chick flick" with me snuggled on the couch – he always puts us first no matter how busy he gets.

Closing thoughts:

I love our story. I love that Patrick is so passionate about hormones and the irony that we have four girls! We have a new legacy of mommas. I'm thankful and grateful for what God has given me: my husband, my children and to be a part of this story that has come to change so many people's lives. It's overwhelming.

Daily, I'm on my knees praying for my husband and The

Wellness Way. We are on a quest to continue the relentless pursuit of doing the right thing and getting the information out to the people. We will continue regardless of what comes our way; regardless of the hate mail and regardless of obstacles.

One of the biggest lessons I've learned and wish to pass on to you, dear reader: Don't let your future be dictated by someone else's fear.

Patty's Story

After 11 years of infertility, exploratory surgeries and rounds of IVF, I was feeling done. It was hard wanting to be pregnant, seeing pregnant strangers or being with a friend who was expecting a baby. I had been told by the IVF doctors I'd never be able to carry a baby in my womb. They told me I would have to look into a surrogate or adopt. I wanted to have a hysterectomy. If I couldn't use my female organs, I didn't want them.

When we had found The Wellness Way and Dr. Patrick, a cancelation enabled us to get in right away. I knew it was meant to be!

We learned a whole new lifestyle at The Wellness Way. The approach was completely different. From all that we learned, I have referred my sister, a neighbor, people with cancer and those with other health challenges. While some people are opposed to trying anything different, others have great results with The Wellness Way.

We had several people who were skeptical and told us it wouldn't work. I faced my own challenge. I worked in the dairy industry. Due to my allergies, I had to eliminate dairy from my diet. I often heard "don't bite the hand that feeds you;" but I had to do what was right for my body.

We are now expecting our second baby and weren't even trying – it just happened. We weren't trying but we also weren't not trying. We figured since it took 11 years to have our son, he would be our only child. Then I started waking up with nausea and wasn't feeling well. I was 8 weeks along before I realized I was pregnant.

When I share my Wellness Way story, a lot of people are concerned about insurance coverage. I tell them all it's worth it. If this is what you want, and this is your dream in life, then there really is no dollar amount. When we went through IVF, we spent tens of thousands of dollars. All the medications were out of pocket as well. When I talked to my insurance company about the IVF, I was told having a child isn't a necessity of life and they wouldn't cover it. Now, I tell people to put that money toward fixing your body the right way. Let it work the way it should and treat it right. You only have one body.

Amanda's Story

I had been pretty healthy in my teen years. I had no challenges with my cycles. Everything seemed just fine. The challenges started after I decided to go off my birth control – Depo-Provera injections.

I struggled with stage IV endometriosis and cysts for about 10 years. I felt like I lived a double life. With endometriosis I looked like every other happy and healthy person on the outside. However, at home I spent most of my time with a heating pad and on high doses of pain medication. I hated to tell anyone how I was feeling. I often felt like I was viewed as broken or just making up the symptoms. Endometriosis is a very lonely disease. It drained me both physically and mentally. I felt like a burden causing my family to miss out on so many opportunities. My husband was very supportive and stayed by my side through it all.

I tried every medication to the maximum limits – even to the point of signing waiver forms for these higher doses – had my uterus scraped yearly and was in a hopeless situation. During one emergency surgery, the doctor thought the challenge was my appendix and removed it. My appendix was actually fine. I felt like an experiment to the doctors I was seeing.

Everything we tried seemed to work for a month or so before the pain returned full force. The doctors had no more answers or treatments to try. We were out of options, except for a drastic hysterectomy, and even then, I couldn't be guaranteed a pain free life. All the courses of action we had taken had damaged my body more than helped. I am still challenged with some of the side effects of the drugs I had been given.

I found myself at my chiropractor's office, desperate for help. I was ready to try anything. When my chiropractor reached out to Dr. Patrick to consult, he looked at my tests and asked if I was a 60-year-old woman in menopause. I was a 31-year-old woman. After starting my Wellness Way journey, I was pain free after 3 months! My chiropractor was so impacted, he became a Wellness Way affiliate, so he would be able to help others.

I haven't had any medication or surgery in over two years and I'm not looking back now. In fact, I would be afraid to go back to my previous doctor-the one who "accidently" took out my appendix. I'm afraid I would be kicked out for how strongly I feel about my health and the hope The Wellness Way has restored in my life.

It wasn't always easy, but you must to do the right thing for your health. I have a supportive husband, but still had a lot of criticism from those who didn't understand what I was doing and choosing. I had to choose to stay the course and do the right thing for my family, for my health.

I share my story hoping that it helps others find the help they need at The Wellness Way. I don't want anyone to have to go through the life of pain and misery, so many health challenges can cause, especially in the way of female hormones. I feel better at 33 then I did in my 20's. Thanks to The Wellness Way Approach I have my life back, and I know they can do that for so many more people!

Joy's Story

I had been a healthy young woman until I went off the Depo-Provera injections I was using as birth control. The years leading up to our Wellness Way journey had been filled with tons of attempts to finding natural remedies to balance my hormones and tons of frustration and disappointment with each one. I was almost 30-years-old. My husband and I had been married for 10 years. By this time, we had a miscarriage and lost twins. I was heartbroken and losing hope of having children.

To top things off, I had just had my adrenal function tested and was told I'd be on medication for the rest of my life.

From the moment we walked into The Wellness Way and

our first appointment with Dr. Patrick, things were different. He was so upbeat and positive, even after we shared the adrenal test results with him. This was the first time I'd ever seen a doctor upbeat or positive after looking at my situation. To be honest, this was what gave me hope to continue on. In fact, during our first appointment he said, "Give me six months, and you'll be pregnant!" How could I not have hope?

Well, sure enough, we had our first baby girl in 2009! We were so excited when we conceived our first miracle. You can only imagine our surprise and amazement when three months later we conceived our second baby girl! Fifteen months after our second daughter was born, we conceived our son.

Not only was Dr. Patrick invaluable in helping us start our family, but with two babies so close together, and a third shortly after you can only imagine all the hormone fluctuations. He was an amazing help through the breastfeeding, post-partum care and nearly back to back pregnancies. And those adrenals? No problem.

One thing I can say about Dr. Patrick, when he gets your hormones where they need to be, they work just fine!

Erin's Story

My family started seeing Dr. Patrick at The Wellness Way when two of our three daughters had adverse reactions to childhood vaccines.

Two years later, I noticed a lump in my breast. I was 32-years-old. The first thing I did was call The Wellness Way. I was able to see Dr. Patrick immediately. To say I was anxious is an understatement. The Wellness Way is a fantastic community. When you walk in the door, you know you are in good hands. While I was meeting with Dr. Patrick, one of the front desk associates took two of my young daughters, so I could have a focused discussion. The first thing Dr. Patrick did was help me calm down. After an exam, he had me schedule an appointment with my OB/GYN to order a mammogram and ultrasound. He assured me he was confident I would be told the cyst was benign. He said they would watch it over the next several years. Dr. Patrick went on to ask a few more questions. By the time I left that first appointment, I felt much more confident.

The next appointment with my OB/GYN went as Dr. Patrick predicted. She did a quick breast exam, ordered the mammogram and ultrasound. During that time of waiting for appointments, our family had other visits with Dr. Patrick. Each time he would give me pieces of information to research. He already knew what I was going to face and wanted to prepare me. His confidence calmed me and my husband immeasurably.

Immediately after the mammogram, I was taken for additional testing. After a few days, I received a phone call. I was told the cyst was benign and they would keep an eye on it. I went back to Dr. Patrick armed with my good news. His answer was simple. I was "safe" for now, but my estrogen levels were abnormally high. I had a choice to make. I could either let things go and in 3-5 years I'd most likely be facing a cancer diagnosis with 3 young daughters and a husband in my mid-thirties. Or, I could work to get healthy now. It was an easy decision. Let's do this and get healthy! The date was October 17.

Dr. Patrick laid out the plan for me. I would have a very

restricted diet for six months and the first few weeks would be especially intense. At the end of six months, I'd feel like a whole different woman. I was also excited at the prospect of losing the extra 40 pounds I was carrying. I had recently met a young woman about my age at church who had won her battle with breast cancer. I asked her what she knew about estrogen fed cysts and breast cancer. She pointed at her now flat chest and hair freshly grown back and told me she wished she had known more.

Remember that restricted diet and the date? The very next day was my daughter's birthday. I chose to give her a healthy momma and not have a piece of cake; and for the daughter who had a birthday two weeks later; and the next daughter, 3 days after the second. I said "no" to unhealthy eating at Thanksgiving, Christmas and all the holiday gatherings; including New Years, Valentine's Day, my husband's birthday and our wedding anniversary. Finally, six months later, on my birthday I was able to indulge in a piece of fruit. Dr. Patrick was and is right. Food is emotional. Your health is largely dictated by the eating choices you make.

I had a lot of questions from family and friends. I didn't want sympathy. I didn't need critics. This was an intentional decision to give my children a healthy mother, my husband a healthy wife and to reclaim my health. I cut out all sugar and nearly all my favorite foods. I learned a lesson that would affect many decisions we would make for health in the coming years. I was able to teach my beautiful daughters what has now become a family mantra – "food is fuel, not a friend". Was it hard? Yes! Was it worth it? Undoubtedly.

I've not been back to the OB/GYN for the last 10 ½ years. Why? The cyst dissolved, and had I followed their advice, I wouldn't be where I am today. My husband may have been a single father with three young daughters. I didn't want to play their guess and wait game. There was too much at stake.

For any woman wondering if taking care of herself and/or her hormones is worth it – absolutely. Look at your children, look at your husband. Get over the "hard" and do the hard and right thing. There's too much life to live. Choose to live it.

Brenda's Story

Dr. Patrick has been instrumental in helping me understand the proper approach to healthcare instead of our current system. I met him after dealing with a health problem that had me seeing several doctors and specialists, visiting many emergency rooms, and on an overall path that was leading me down a spiral toward further disease and illness. I was honestly starting to wonder how much longer I could function at my current lifestyle pace. I felt like I was starting to lose my grip on my reality.

He is passionate about his calling. It was evident from the first time I met him. He took time to understand my story and concerns, ordered labs, and offered key nutritional changes that identified the underlying cause of my condition and allowed my body to take the steps needed for proper healing. He is an absolute visionary when it comes to the immune system, hormones, and understanding the biological root cause behind the symptoms. He helped me pull the pieces of the puzzle together and empowered me to take control to create a path that I didn't even know existed.

Dr. Patrick is also a genius at the biochemistry involved at the intersection between stress and illness. My life has been transformed by the knowledge of how stress impacts my hormones. This understanding has helped me slow the chatter of mind and pace of my life by giving me the ability to witness and understand the biological response to stressful situations. He helped me understand the chemicals involved in stress and the damage that can result to my hormones and body. I was able to see for the first time that my power lies in my response to any situation or perceived problem. I can control the stress reaction by simply becoming aware of it. I came to him with a health problem that he not only helped me restore but he also helped me find my power. Talk about transformation! I am beyond fortunate to have him in my life and am honored to be able to watch him change the lives of those around me.

Nicole's Story

So many things are clear when looking back. Hindsight is definitely 20/20. Since puberty, I have struggled with my periods. In high school they were regular in terms of time, but they were also painful leading to missed school. I also struggled with anemia so severe I was seeing specialists, and having colonoscopies to find the source of low iron levels. These specialists never found the cause of the anemia and why I would frequently pass out. I now understand my periods were way too heavy and I was losing too much blood.

My mom approved the use of birth control to help steady my period. I did find some relief for the couple of years that I was on it. I left for college and started planning a wedding. I knew that my periods were inconsistent. I wanted to have a more regular life and let my body adjust, find a normal rhythm. I knew this would take some time so 6 months before my husband and I got married, I went off birth control.

After stopping the birth control, I went months without getting a period. I was a virgin at the time, but I was convinced I had somehow gotten pregnant. When it did come it was incredibly painful and it would then be months before having another one.

I finally went to see a Nurse Practitioner about the issues. She did some further testing and I was diagnosed with Polycystic Ovary Syndrome (PCOS). Because I had such irregular periods, they told me it would likely be very difficult for me to conceive. This news was devastating. I found out a few months before I was supposed to get married. I had the conversation with my fiancé. I knew he had always wanted to have children.

"I don't know if I'm going to be able to have kids. Are you sure you still want to marry me even if this is something I can't give you?" I asked him. He was surprised but said whatever it takes, we'll figure this out together.

When I was younger and had gone on mission trips, one thing they asked us during team building exercises was our biggest fear. My biggest fear was always that I wouldn't be able to have kids. When we were going through pre-marital counseling, I said I didn't want kids. I think it was a defense mechanism. I believed that if I didn't want children, it wouldn't be painful to find out that I couldn't. Through that pre-marital counseling, I realized that I really did want kids. The reality that I might be unable to have children felt like a nightmare.

We started our marriage in this stage of not knowing what our future family would look like. During that first year of marriage while dealing with the diagnosis of PCOS, I gained

70 pounds. When we had been married two years, I was still in college, so we weren't actively trying to have a baby. Because I knew that the possibility existed that it would be difficult for me to conceive, we decided we weren't going to prevent any pregnancy with birth control. We decided that if it happens, it happens. A baby would be God's gift to us. Reality was, all these people around me were getting pregnant that didn't want to get pregnant. I was having a hard time processing our situation. We were married. We had a good home for welcoming babies. Why wasn't this happening for us? I went into a depression thinking parenthood was never going to happen for us.

One night I was just lying in bed and I started praying. *"God, I do feel like I'm going to have a baby someday, but could you give me a dream or a sign or something to get my mind in the right mindset if adoption is my future? Please bring me some sort of clarity. I'm afraid of the unknown."* That night I dreamed I was in a dark room with my eyes closed, rubbing my belly and feeling that distinct kick of a baby growing in the womb. I felt in my dream that someone had said, "His name is Simon." I woke up wondering what it meant. Simon is very specific and a name I wouldn't normally have picked for a baby. However, God has named a lot of people throughout history. I looked up the meaning of the name Simon; *He has heard.* I was stunned. The next month I found out I was pregnant with my son. Of course, we named him Simon!

After Simon was born, I was still very overweight. My doctor prescribed Metformin, a prescription often given to people who have PCOS. It helps insulin resistance, a common concern with PCOS. It gave me digestive upset. I never knew when I would have diarrhea and it was awful.

After a month, I stopped taking the Metformin and decided I was going to have to live with the situation and deal with it. I felt like at this time, God was whispering to me, "get your body back to healthy and the second one will come." I tried everything. Exercising. Drinking meal replacement shakes. Eating healthy. I was doing all I knew to do. You know the standard to get your body healthy-diet and exercise. I lost 20 pounds on my own, but it was difficult.

While all of this was happening, I was struggling with an auto-immune condition that no one could identify. I had eczema all over my body. After I had Simon, the eczema got worse. One night, I cried myself to sleep. My body was on fire. My husband was draping wet towels all over me. It was the only thing that offered even a bit of soothing relief. We started considering moving to Florida because tanning seemed to help with the Vitamin D. I had all these things I was trying to piece together, and I just couldn't. When I was 23, I was diagnosed with Rheumatoid Arthritis. I was in my junior year of nursing school and I could not write notes because it hurt my joints so badly. I got myself an iPad and laptop to do everything I could digitally. Holding a pencil was way too much.

I was overweight. I had this terrible bleeding eczema all over my body. I had tried everything. I had used steroids. I tried Chinese medicine. I tried silver. If I thought it would help eczema, I bought it. I spent thousands of dollars. Some remedies might help for a short time, but if I ever went a day without it, the symptoms would creep right back.

I was exercising and eating healthy, but not losing the weight. I found a detox program online. I decided since I'd heard a lot of people lose a lot of weight on detox, I bought it.

The program was a 21-day detox, where you take some supplements and they tell you what to eat every single day. At the end of the detox, the end of the 3 weeks, I was finally seeing some relief for the first time in my life from the eczema. It was almost gone. It was interesting because I wasn't doing anything topically. I didn't realize it, I was just working on my gut and my insides. Two weeks later I had a period for the first time in months. Two weeks after that I conceived my daughter. During pregnancy your immune system is suppressed so things tend to go better for those with auto-immune challenges. After I had my daughter, I was thinking *"ok, there is something to this detox thing."*

As a nurse working in labor and delivery, I was used to the medical mindset and pharmacology practices. I was stuck with the mindset of taking a drug for a condition. I didn't like the drugs they gave me; often they made me feel worse. I couldn't find anything else that would work. I thought I was stuck.

I remembered the eczema had gone away with the detox. I was starting to connect the dots. However, I felt like I couldn't be living in a state of detox all the time. I went to a conference. The man who had created the detox was there. I asked him about the idea of living in a state of detox. He told me it was possible. There are ways to support your body through supplementation to keep the inflammation at bay. Inflammation. There was another dot. I did another detox and felt fantastic. This was the only time I'd lose weight quickly and the eczema would go away. I was doing research and found there was a connection between eczema and gut health. There's something to this gut health thing. I was determined to get healthy.

I've always been transparent about my journey on

Facebook. One day, someone reached out to me and told me about this gut protocol and invited me to do it with them. It was a thousand-dollar program plus the supplements. I was desperate. While I was doing this gut healing program, someone else reached out to me and asked if I'd ever heard of Dr. Patrick and The Wellness Way. I was in the middle of the program. I had spent over $1000 on this gut thing; I was going to stick with it. They were relentless "he really makes the connections when he talks about your gut health, he talks about how it affects your hormones, inflammation, everything." All I could think was it's *all* connected! It's not just gut = eczema, it's gut = hormones and eczema and I have all these things going on. Maybe it all originates in my gut!

I was seeing some results from the gut protocol, but not like I wanted for how much I had paid. I called The Wellness Way and set an appointment with Dr. Patrick. I remember sitting in the waiting room thinking *"Either these people are going to be a bunch of weirdos and totally out there or there's going to be something to this. I'm about to find out."* They took my x-rays and showed me the inflammation in my gut. *They showed me the inflammation in my gut. Dots connected.* I talked with Dr. Patrick and told him my story. I had brought in my giant tub of supplements that I was taking. His response, "there's nothing wrong with these supplements but how do you know they are the ones you need?" All I could say was, "I don't know, it's just part of the protocol." He showed me the problem with the protocol. It wasn't individualized to each person. That's why I wasn't getting the results I was looking for. He started to help me shift my mind and think differently. I went to the Inflammation Talk the next day. Finally, it clicked. The Wellness Way Clinics offer

Inflammation Talks every couple of weeks for new patients. This talk is the foundation and introduces new patients to The Wellness Way Approach. Inflammation is the key to all sources of disease and dysfunction within the body. This is what I had been looking for. I had been researching for years trying to find answers and connect the dots between my gut, eczema, auto-immune conditions and PCOS. I finally found someone who could put those connections together!

After the Inflammation Talk, I boldly approached Dr. Patrick. The only thing I could think was, *"if there's anything I am going to do, I have to work for this guy. I have to learn everything he knows."* I said, "I don't know if you remember me. I was in as a new patient yesterday. I had mentioned that I am a nurse. Your Inflammation Talk opened my eyes. I finally get it. Women's hormones and autoimmune conditions are my passion; it's something I have struggled with. I really think this approach could apply to infertility for women across the country and I want to be an expert. Would you consider bringing me on board?" His response was quick, "Yes, come in for an interview." I was totally blown away. "REALLY?" I'm not typically that bold, but there was something inside me. I knew I couldn't leave without addressing it.

I went in for the interview. The timing was perfect. The Wellness Way Green Bay was looking for a nurse to help with the IV center. It was a great way to get trained and see what happens at The Wellness Way. My Wellness Way journey began. I recognized the difference between The Wellness Way Approach and the traditional medical model. The allopathic medical model sees a list of symptoms and comes up with a diagnosis to treat. They don't look at the whole picture. It didn't resonate with me that I'd have to live a life constantly relying on medication or supplements like others suggested. I felt like I should be able to fix it. Medication or supplements should be part time. The Wellness Way looks at your symptoms, connects them to one or two single root causes to support so you can live in a world of wellness. I was properly tested; my thyroid, hormone and food allergy test.

My food allergy test was eye opening. I discovered I had 42 food allergies. To this day, I have not had anyone come in to the Green Bay clinic with more than me. I started eliminating those immediately. It was very difficult, but necessary. I started taking a few supplements to help with my gut, my iron deficiency and to balance my hormones. Unlike a traditional PCOS patient, I had very low testosterone. A lot of the protocol used in the medical world wouldn't have worked for me; I wouldn't have known why if I hadn't gotten my hormones tested as thoroughly as The Wellness Way does. Within a month of following The Wellness Way Approach, I got my period for the first time in months. It was the first normal period in my life. From then on, I would get it every single month. The first week I lost 10 pounds. I was 80 pounds overweight at that time. Within my first two months I lost over 25 pounds and 80 pounds within the first 6 months. I was feeling like myself again. I had more vitality and energy. Within two months my eczema was completely gone. I was a walking testimony to The Wellness Way Approach!

Everyone had told me I would have auto-immune conditions and take steroids the rest of my life. The Rheumatoid Arthritis, eczema, weight and PCOS were three different systems that were all broken. When I came to The Wellness Way I realized they were connected; they weren't isolated instances. I started sharing my Wellness Way testimony with my friends and have become a great referral source. I soaked up everything I could about hormones and how to balance the body. When my husband and I decided we were ready, we conceived baby #3 the first time we tried. I believe this lifestyle is for everyone. You shouldn't have to take supplements or medication for the rest of your life. Your body can be whole, well, and free of conditions as long as you know and avoid your triggers. That's what makes The Wellness Way unique.

My dreams and desires to reach as many people as I can are becoming a reality. At The Wellness Way, we don't have specialties; everything within the body is connected. However, I have been able to build a practice around this one very special focus. It is so much fun to help women find the root cause of their issues, and then watch them feel so much better like I did. We've had people reach out from all over the world through the power of social media. Women from Switzerland, Argentina, Bhutan, Asia, England, have found answers through The Wellness Way.

Every time I share The Wellness Way message, I tell my patients, "you are not broken." A lot of times when women are not able to conceive, it devastates them. It's part of their womanhood; they feel like they are broken. Your body is responding to your environment, we just have to figure out why and fix it. You were created to have babies if that is what you want!

FINAL THOUGHTS

So, here we are. The end of the book. What now? Well, one thing is for certain. You know how I feel about several issues.

Infertility

Hormone Challenges either not being addressed properly or being misdiagnosed as psychological problems.

Divorce

Unhappy marriages

Heart disease

Diabetes

Cancer

I will keep speaking out and sharing the message of The Wellness Way clinics and a hope for real health instead of just an accepted diagnosis. But the real question is, *what are you going to do?*

So, I want to ask you, did you learn something? Do you think a little differently? What are your next steps? Find a Wellness Way clinic near you. The only way we can get you the care you need, is to test you. We don't guess what you need, we test to find what you need. Even if we have helped a friend or family member close to you, we can't just do the same thing for you. You are a different and unique person. *You* need to get tested to figure out what *you* need.

Unless you take action, you are going to be in the same boat as the rest of the population-sick and miserable. I've laid out some very practical steps in your *To Do Lists*. These will help. A lot. However, if there is an underlying hormone issue, which there typically is, they will only get you so far. Without a doubt, one thing I hope you take away from this book is not to leave your health in an uncertain state.

Don't guess. Get tested. It's that simple. Any Wellness Way Clinic can help you with that. In fact, you can even go on our website and get our favorite hormone test for yourself. We want to provide you with the information you need to take the next steps. But now you need to take those steps yourself. There is so much to gain and nothing to lose. Except your health, if you do not.

www.thewellnesswayclinics.com/hormone-test/
www.thewellnesswayclinics.com/clinics/

Yours in Health,

QUESTIONS FOR SELF-REFLECTION:

If I were to rate my health on a scale of 1-5 I would be:

Have I been struggling with hormone challenges?

Are there other areas of my own health and wellness that I believe can be handled better in my life?

Given the Zones laid out for me, do I feel like my cycle is normal?

Am I willing to stay on the current wellness track I've been on?

Is becoming a happier and healthier version of myself something I am willing to take action on?

Am I willing to seek out a Wellness Way Clinic to have my hormones tested?

If I were to rate my marriage/relationship on a scale of 1-5 we would be:

How am I doing on the *To Do Lists* for my spouse?

What can I do right away to help make a positive change?

Am I okay with the fact that my spouse has a different cycle than I do, that we are physiologically different?

Am I willing to support and help my spouse take the next steps to have their hormones tested if I believe there may be an underlying health concern?

Dr. Patrick Flynn

_____

_____

_____

_____

_____

_____

_____

_____

_____

_____

_____

_____

_____

_____

QUESTIONS TO DISCUSS WITH YOUR SPOUSE:

On a scale of 1-5 where would you rate my health?

After looking at the Zones, do you feel like my cycle is normal?

Would you support me in seeking out a Wellness Way Clinic to have my hormones tested?

On a scale of 1-5 where would you rate our marriage/ relationship?

How am I doing on your *To Do List*?

Which areas do you feel I do really well in?

What items on your *To Do List* do I need to improve upon?

Are you willing to have your hormones tested so that we can make sure we are both healthy as we do life and grow old together?

_____

_____

_____

_____

_____

_____

_____

_____

_____

_____

_____

_____

_____

_____

RECIPE SECTION

We all know that food has a close tie to our emotions. We also know that food is either healing or harming to you. The Wellness Way recommends eating only organic foods. Conventionally grown and processed foods are inflammatory and should be avoided. Some foods such as maca root powder, cacao, and organic raw nuts may be easier to buy online if you are unable to find them at a local grocery store. We put together a few recipes that can help you not only keep your hormones balanced but may also help you prepare a memorable date night in for you and your spouse. Cooking together can really heat things up! There are so many foods listed, the possibilities are endless, but here are a few favorites. Remember to avoid any food allergies you may have. Bon Appétit!

Foods to focus on for hormone support:

Organic Fruits:
Avocados
Figs
Pomegranate
Raspberries
Mangoes
Citrus
Strawberries

Organic Vegetables:
Celery
Dark leafy greens, especially arugula, kale and spinach
Asparagus
Beets
Artichokes

Organic Grass-Fed meats, Wild Game
and Wild Caught Sea Food
Wild caught Salmon (farm raised salmon is highly inflammatory!)
Tuna
Shellfish
Lamb
Wild game

Organic Spices, Organic Fresh Herbs
Chili peppers
Fresh herbs
Fennel

Saffron
Fenugreek
Ginger
Cinnamon
Vanilla
Ginseng
Cacao – raw, not cocoa or chocolate
Maca
Ashwagandha
Roses

Additional Proteins and Fats:
Organic Free-Range Eggs
Organic Raw Almonds
Organic Raw Brazil Nuts

Organic Beverages:
Coffee
Organic herbal teas made with above spices and herbs

Sweeteners:
Raw unfiltered locally sourced honey
Hardwood sourced xylitol

Morning Starters or Mid-day Pick-ups:

Smooth As Silk Smoothie
1 cup organic non-dairy milk, preferably almond
½ cup organic coconut water or coconut cream for thicker more pudding like consistency
½ cup organic blueberries or strawberries
1 organic banana
1 tsp organic raw maca powder
1 Tbsp organic raw cacao nibs
1 Tbsp melted organic raw cacao butter
Ice cubes to desired consistency.

Blend all ingredients except cacao butter together, once well blended, slowly stir in cacao butter and serve. Double the recipe and serve to your loved one for bonus points!

Berry Sexy Smoothie
1 cup organic nondairy milk, preferably almond
½ cup pomegranate seeds
½ cup organic blueberries or strawberries
1 organic banana
½ organic avocado
1 tsp organic raw cacao powder

Blend all ingredients together and serve.

Get Your Motor Running Coffee
Pour your usual size coffee mug leaving room for:
1 ½ tsp organic raw cacao powder
2 Tbsp organic coconut or organic almond milk
Desired amount of raw unfiltered honey
½ tsp organic cinnamon or ginger
1 tsp organic raw maca powder

A milk frother blends this well right in your cup!

Snacks and Sweet Bites:

Dark Chocolate Cherry Love bites
8 pitted medjool dates, chopped and soaked in hot water for 15 minutes
2-3 Tbsp filtered water as needed for consistency
1/3 cup organic dried cherries
¾ cup organic raw almonds or Brazil nuts
½ cup organic raw cashews
1/3 cup organic raw cacao powder
1 tsp organic raw maca powder
1/8-1/4 tsp sea salt or Himalayan pink salt
1 tsp organic vanilla

In a powerful blender or food processor, blend almonds, cashews, cacao powder, maca, salt, vanilla until fine.
Add the dates, cherries slowly while processing, scraping sides and adding water as needed.
Roll tablespoon size servings into balls.
Roll balls into raw cacao powder
Store in container in refrigerator or freezer

Va-Va-Vanilla Roasted Nuts
2 cups organic raw almonds or Brazil nuts
2/3 cup xylitol*
¼ cup filtered water
1 tsp organic vanilla extract
Pinch of sea salt.

Place almonds on a baking sheet lined with parchment paper. Toast almonds briefly at 350*. They'll get a second toasting later, so don't over toast at this point.

In a frying pan, bring xylitol, water, vanilla and salt to a boil and continue to boil for one minute.

Add your nuts to the frying pan and stir continuously until all the liquid has evaporated. Continue stirring just a little longer for the xylitol to caramelize a little – they can go from a little caramelized to burnt very quickly, so keep stirring!

Pour nuts onto the parchment paper from earlier to cool. Remember, they were just in boiling sugar, they are hot! Don't try to separate them with your fingers.

Have fun with the recipe and change up the spices and flavors. Add organic cinnamon, chili, cardamom or saffron.

Love Bites
2 Tbsp organic raw maca
3 Tbsp raw organic cacao powder
¾ cup organic nut butter of choice
½ cup organic tahini
½ cup raw unfiltered honey
¼ cup of any one of: organic raisins, dried cherries, cacao nibs, crushed nuts
Cacao for dusting or cacao ganache for dipping fondue style.

Combine ingredients in a bowl and stir until well combined. Roll into bit size balls.

Chocolate Ganache
1 cup raw organic cacao butter
½ cup organic maple syrup, raw unfiltered honey, organic coconut syrup or similar organic liquid sweetener
½ cup organic raw cacao powder
1 tsp organic vanilla
Gently melt, stirring to incorporate completely. Done! Use as a dip for fondue with any of the listed fruits, or for any of the snack balls listed above. Also make a yummy frosting.

Chocolate bark
Whip up a batch of chocolate ganache, add an assortment of dried fruits or nuts. Pour mixture onto parchment lined baking sheet and place in fridge or freezer to harden. Once hardened, break into pieces and store in an airtight container in the fridge.

For more dessert recipes check out www.thewellnesswayclinics.com for a free e-book filled with healthy desserts!

Condiments:

Maca-mole!
2-3 organic avocados diced/mashed
Juice from one organic lime
½ organic red onion diced
1 small organic tomato diced
2 tsp organic raw maca
Sea Salt, fresh cilantro, jalapeno and a dash of chili powder
to taste
Mix and enjoy with any organic raw veggies.

Creamy Avocado Sauce
1 organic avocado
1 cup organic fresh basil
½ cup organic fresh cilantro
2 organic green onions
½ tsp organic minced garlic
¼ cup organic tahini
Juice of 1 organic lime
2 tsp organic raw maca powder
Pink Himalayan Salt and organic pepper to taste

Combine ingredients in food processor. Doubling the recipe
right away isn't a bad idea. You'll want to use this as a con-
diment on everything! Thin with water to create a fresh and
creamy salad dressing.

Spicy Ginger Masala
Grind together:
1 piece of organic ginger root equivalent to 1 tsp
5 organic green onions peeled
2 teaspoons organic coconut flakes
1 tsp organic peppercorns
2 tsp organic cumin seeds
1 tsp organic raw maca powder
½ tsp organic fennel seeds

Add water as needed to create a smooth paste.
Use as a rub or seasoning to any meat you desire.

Entrees:

Pan Seared Wild Salmon
Desired number of Wild Salmon fillets
About 2 Tbsp organic avocado oil for each pan you will be frying

Wash salmon fillets and pat dry
Before you add the oil, preheat the pan a bit, this will also help the salmon from sticking without smoking up the house!
Place fillets skin side up in a lightly greased (coconut or avocado oil) frying pan over medium heat
Gently shake the pan so the fillets won't stick – but don't splash that hot oil!
After about 7-10 minutes, you'll see a distinct line in the middle of the fillet, now is the time to gently flip.
Turn off the heat, I know, it's not done yet. Trust me. Cover the frying pan and let that salmon finish by steaming for an additional 10 minutes for medium, 12-13 minutes for medium-well.
Serving suggestion: serve with roasted asparagus and Creamy Avocado Sauce

Spicy Lamb Meatballs
Preheat oven to 400*
**Lamb can be substituted for any other organic grass-fed ground meat or wild game.
1-pound organic grass-fed ground lamb
½ tsp organic ginger powder

½ tsp organic cinnamon
½ tsp organic oregano
½ tsp organic black pepper
½ tsp organic garam masala
Add all ingredients into mixing bowl and mix thoroughly. Divide into about 18 balls. Place onto a lightly greased baking sheet and cook for about 15 minutes or until internal temperature reaches 165*
Serving Suggestion: serve with arugula or spinach salad with figs and pomegranate arils

Smokey Garlic Shrimp
¼ cup organic avocado or organic coconut oil
3 organic garlic cloves minced
1 ½ pounds peeled wild shrimp
1 teaspoon organic smoked paprika
¾ teaspoon organic ground cumin
Pinch of organic saffron
Organic lemon slices

Heat oil in a large skillet over medium-low heat. Add garlic. When garlic is golden, stir in shrimp and spices. Continue to cook about 5-10 minutes until shrimp is pink, turning them twice in that time. Once the shrimp is plated, squeeze one lemon slice over each dish.
Serving suggestion: serve on a bed of arugula or spinach either fresh or lightly wilted

One more recipe of interest:

Coconut oil Body Butter Recipe
½ cup organic virgin coconut oil
½ cup shea butter
1 tsp grapeseed oil
5 drops essential oil of your choice
Mix all ingredients together either in a bowl with a whisk or
in a food processor until airy consistency.
Store in a glass airtight container.
Enjoy!